Practical Aspects of ECG Recording

Jacqui Crawford
Linda Doherty

Practical Aspects of ECG Recording
Jacqui Crawford
Linda Doherty

ISBN: 978-1-905539-30-7

First published 2012

British Library Cataloguing in Publication Data

A catalogue record for this book is available from the British Library

Notice

Clinical practice and medical knowledge constantly evolve. Standard safety precautions must be followed, but, as knowledge is broadened by research, changes in practice, treatment and drug therapy may become necessary or appropriate. Readers must check the most current product information provided by the manufacturer of each drug to be administered and verify the dosages and correct administration, as well as contraindications. It is the responsibility of the practitioner, utilising the experience and knowledge of the patient, to determine dosages and the best treatment for each individual patient. Any brands mentioned in this book are as examples only and are not endorsed by the publisher. Neither the publisher nor the authors assume any liability for any injury and/or damage to persons or property arising from this publication.

To contact M&K Publishing write to:

M&K Update Ltd · The Old Bakery · St. John's Street

Keswick · Cumbria CA12 5AS

Tel: 01768 773030 · Fax: 01768 781099

publishing@mkupdate.co.uk

www.mkupdate.co.uk

Designed and typeset by Mary Blood

Printed in England by Ferguson Print, Keswick

Practical Aspects of ECG Recording

Other books from M&K include

The ECG Workbook 2/e
ISBN: 9781905539772

Cardiac Arrhythmia Recognition: An easy learning guide
ISBN: 97819055395536

Routine Blood Results Explained 2/e
ISBN: 97819055395383

Arterial Blood Gas Analysis: An easy learning guide
ISBN: 97819055395048

Haemodynamic Monitoring & Manipulation: An easy learning guide
ISBN: 97819055395468

Research Issues in Health and Social Care
ISBN: 9781905539208

A Pre-Reader for the Foundation Degree in Health and Social Care Practice
ISBN: 9781905539680

Preoperative Assessment & Perioperative Management
ISBN: 9781905539024

Ward Based Critical Care: A guide for health professionals
ISBN: 9781905539024

Contents

Figures

Tables

Preface

Practical Aspects of ECG Recording is for everyone who records or teaches ECGs. As cardiorespiratory educators we get frequent requests for good sources of information on how to record ECGs. However, most electrocardiography courses and textbooks skim over recording and place their main emphasis on interpretation. The purpose of this book is to shift the focus firmly back onto good recording technique as the fundamental starting point for developing ECG competency.

We are passionate about improving patient quality of care and safety particularly in relation to the recording of routine diagnostic tests. Whilst interpretation skills are vital, it is easy to forget that correctly recording an ECG is just as crucial for accurate interpretation and understanding of the interpretative process.

It is estimated that billions of ECGs are recorded worldwide every year and studies indicate up to 84 % of these may be recorded incorrectly. This can lead to misdiagnosis, inappropriate treatment and care. Not only does poor recording technique put the patient at risk, it also undermines the reputation of both the profession involved and the organisation they work for. *Practical Aspects of ECG Recording*, explores and demonstrates the knowledge and skills required to produce diagnostic quality ECGs. Whilst this book can be read as a theoretical text, it is intended to be used in conjunction with a hands-on practical ECG training course, clinical experience and reflective practice.

The 14 chapters provide useful learning opportunities for practitioners at all levels of experience. The contents have been specifically designed to develop the reader's knowledge, practical skills and behaviours in ECG recording which are directly applicable to everyday clinical practice. Simple facts are included as the foundations on which to develop the more complex concepts and explanations, often with the help of figures, photographs and tables which provide visual reinforcement, clarification and support of the text. As the book progresses the reader is exposed to all aspects of recording from the initial patient contact to archiving the final product. Each chapter begins with a set of learning objectives that focus the reader's attention to the information they are expected to attain by the end of the section.

Although the chapters are self-contained, pedagogical aids provide an opportunity to deepen learning through the integration of accumulated skills and knowledge. Each chapter contains review and comprehension questions, and key points which test the reader's understanding, skills and knowledge on newly acquired topic areas. Active learning is encouraged through the use of 'what if' prediction style questions and clinical scenarios which allow the reader to apply critical thinking, reasoning and problem solving skills. Each chapter ends with a summary of the key points. This provides a brief outline of the main concepts and facts discussed providing a revision snapshot of the topic area.

About the Authors

Jacqui Crawford graduated from the University of Ulster with a BSc (Hons) Clinical Science. She was awarded an MSc in Medical Science from the University in 2001. Having worked for twenty years in cardiac and respiratory physiology she was appointed as a Lecturer in Clinical Physiology at the University of Ulster in 2003. She is a fellow of the Society for Cardiovascular Science and Technology. She is currently the Course Director for the BSc (Hons) Clinical Physiology and Healthcare Science and also lectures on these programmes.

Linda Doherty graduated from the University of Ulster with a BSc (Hons) Clinical Science. She was awarded an MSc in Medical Science from the University in 2001. She worked in various clinical areas including cardiology, cardiac surgery, medical and respiratory investigations before being appointed by the University of Ulster as a lecturer in 2002. Linda lectures on both the Clinical Physiology and Healthcare Science programmes. She is a fellow of the Society for Cardiovascular Science and Technology.

Chapter 1

An introduction to electrocardiography

By the end of this chapter you should be able to:
- define a 12-lead electrocardiogram
- identify indications for recording an electrocardiogram
- appreciate the benefit of using a standardised ECG recording approach
- recognise ECG accuracy will always be limited as some events are outside the control of practitioners and current technology.

Since its introduction into clinical practice the electrocardiogram has become one of the most widely available and utilised investigations. ECGs are recorded in a range of settings by practitioners and others involved in fields such as sport and exercise. Despite this there is limited guidance regarding the recording of the electrocardiogram as most textbooks concentrate upon interpretation. Practitioners must be capable of recording accurate ECGs. If skill and experience in electrocardiography is currently not sufficient this can be changed by focusing on and enhancing present practice. The degree to which a practitioner actively engages in continuing professional development and evidence-based practice will be instrumental in determining how quickly these changes occur and ultimately ensure the highest quality healthcare is available for all patients.

What is a 12-lead electrocardiogram?

A 12-lead ECG is a graphical recording obtained by placing ten electrodes on specific positions on the body surface. This provides twelve different views of the electrical activity generated by the myocardium as it depolarises and repolarises to produce the heartbeat. These changes in voltage create a characteristic pattern of positive and negative deflections called waves which can be captured on paper or viewed on a screen. The most frequently seen waves are P, Q, R, S and T; however there are others including F, f, Δ and U waves. Changes in voltage are measured on the vertical axis whilst time is measured on the horizontal axis. This permits the accurate measurement of heart rate, wave durations and timing intervals, wave voltages and the calculation of cardiac axis to be made. Many of these measurements will only be accurate if the electrodes have been placed in precise anatomical positions on the body surface using a standardised methodology. Recording ECGs using a standardised technique permits:

- ECGs recorded at different times, in different settings and by different practitioners to be compared
- changes over time to be monitored
- responses to treatment to be monitored

- accurate comparison with normal reference values to be made and the confident identification of true physiological abnormalities established.

Essentially it is only by using a standardised recording procedure that misdiagnosis due to incorrect electrode placement and/or lead attachment is prevented.

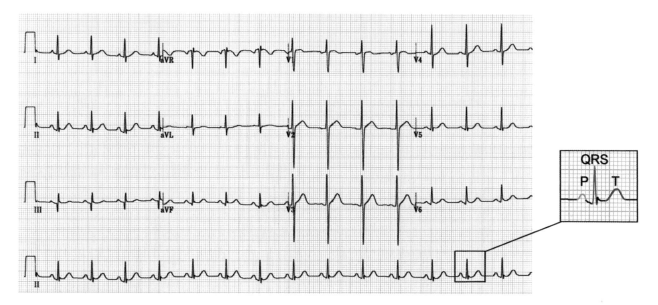

Figure 1.1: Example of a 12-lead ECG highlighting P, QRS complex and T wave.

Indications for recording an electrocardiogram

There are numerous indications for recording an ECG however it is important to understand that the ECG can only directly measure time and voltage; all other information available must be derived or inferred. Research over a number of years has established characteristic patterns and measurements associated with a variety of disease states. However, the sensitivity and specificity of these measurements vary with different pathologies impacting on the ECG's diagnostic value. In other words, the ECG is useful in some situations such as detecting the presence of a myocardial infarction whilst of limited value in others such as determining the extent of non-viable myocardium. An ECG is indicated for:

- the assessment of patients presenting with chest pain
- unexplained dizziness and/or syncope
- the diagnosis and monitoring of cardiovascular disease
- the assessment of therapy outcomes both beneficial and toxic
- presurgical assessment workup
- risk assessment for cardiac disease in individuals with two or more of the following risk factors: diabetes, hypertension, smoking history, obesity, hypercholesterolaemia, strong family history of cardiac disease
- a family history of sudden death
- the assessment of cardiac effects in coexisting systemic disease e.g. renal failure
- monitoring cardiac transplant success or rejection
- adhering to occupational requirements e.g. airline pilots, divers etc.
- epidemiological studies.

There are no absolute contraindications to recording a resting 12-lead ECG in the clinical environment other than in the uncooperative, abusive patient or a patient that refuses to give consent. However in the field ECGs are typically not recorded where privacy and dignity cannot be protected, safety of the patient or practitioner cannot be guaranteed, or it delays transit time to the detriment of overall patient management. Relative contraindications include trauma and the inability to place electrodes correctly on the chest, extensive skin conditions and burns. Screening the general population is not currently recommended.

How accurate is the ECG?

It is important to recognise that a 12-lead ECG is never 100 per cent accurate. Inaccuracy can arise from non-modifiable patient factors such as respiration patterns, post prandial state (period after a meal), gender, race and body habitus. It may also arise from modifiable practitioner factors such as incorrect electrode placement, lead reversal and poor skin preparation. Adhering to guidelines can help limit the extent of inaccuracy and alert the practitioner to ECG changes they may expect in a specific patient. Even when the ECG is recorded strictly to recommendations, a number of limitations still remain. These include:

- **The limited recording period**

ECGs provide data over a specific period in time. In A4 format this equates to approximately ten seconds. Anything that occurs before or after this period is not recorded. For example in the patient complaining of frequent palpitations, it is common to record a normal ECG with no arrhythmias and further tests will be required before a diagnosis can be made. On occasion it is possible to infer a past event may have occurred but it is not possible to be confident. For example the presence of Q waves may indicate an old myocardial infarction with non-viable myocardium. But not all Q waves are indicative of necrosis. They are not seen in all patients with myocardial necrosis and when present are more predictive of inferior than anterior non-viable tissue.

- **False positives and false negatives**

Due to the limited sensitivity and specificity in different disease states, the ECG is prone to producing false positive and false negatives. A false positive occurs when the recorded data indicates a disease or structural change is present when it is not. A false negative suggests that the data is normal in the presence of disease or structural changes. For example a false positive result may occur with ST elevation. In some individuals there is a normal variant called high ST segment take off. This is typically found in young individuals and is not associated with the expected reciprocal ST depression changes or true ischaemic heart disease. The main problem arises when it occurs in the presence of a convincing ischaemic history. Conversely a false negative result may occur in unstable angina. In this case the ECG may be normal yet the patient symptoms represent true ischaemia. Reasons for this include that even with 12 different views of the myocardium there are still electrical blind spots; the expected ST changes can be masked due to pseudonormalisation of the ST/T waves. Pseudonormalisation occurs when abnormal ST/T wave changes revert to a normal pattern. Unless the patient has been monitored or these changes documented at an earlier stage they can be missed. This further highlights the problem that an ECG is a snapshot in time but despite this limitation the ECG remains a cost effective initial diagnostic step in many conditions.

- **Reference values and the definition of normality**

The majority of ECG reference values regarding timing and voltages are based upon limited patient cohorts from the early days of electrocardiography. We now know that there are gender, ethnic, obesity and normal variations. Consequently inaccuracy in interpretation may occur unless interpretation has been made in line with the correct reference values. Consideration must also be made for normal variants to avoid misinterpretation. This may be a particular problem in relation to the athletic heart. Further problems arise when coexisting pathologies are present. For example caution needs to be taken in diagnosing a myocardial infarction (MI) in the presence of left bundle branch block as the aberrant depolarising pathway conceals the acute changes of MI.

- **Day-to-day variability**

Consecutive ECGs are prone to natural variation due to the circadian rhythm, changes in physiological state e.g. nervousness or pain, and even after a meal. Heart rate is the most variable factor, followed by the QT interval. ST segment heights are more stable unless electrodes have been placed in different positions. When comparing serial ECGs, minor changes in waveforms and voltages can be expected.

- **Inter-/intra-observer variability**

ECGs should always be reported by an experienced practitioner. Where computerised interpretation is used the report should be over-read to check for mistakes and omissions. Studies confirm that intra-observer variability in ECG reports (same person reanalysing an ECG) is good. However practitioners do not always agree in their interpretation and inter- observer variability (different individuals analysing the same ECG) is poorer. In theory standardised algorithms applied by the interpretative software packages of ECG machines should overcome the apparent variability. Whilst great improvements in ECG computerised reporting have occurred in recent years, the technology is not fully evolved and will always have to rely on the quality of the data it is fed to analyse.

Although the ECG has many inaccuracies it remains a valuable diagnostic technique. This is because non-modifiable inaccuracies can be accounted for by an experienced practitioner during interpretation and modifiable inaccuracies can be limited by using a standardised ECG recording technique. This allows the ECG to remain an effective and quick diagnostic step in many conditions.

The standardised ECG technique

Papers and textbooks referring to a 'standard 12-lead ECG' often mean that a standard set of leads have been recorded rather than the true full meaning which is a standard set of leads recorded from standard electrode positions at a standard calibration setting. Standardisation was first attempted in the 1930s and continues with the most recent recording guidelines produced by the American Heart Association (2007) and the Society of Cardiological Science and Technology (SCST) endorsed by the British Cardiovascular Society (2010). It is important that all those recording ECGs adhere to the same practice standards in relation to the preparation for and recording of an ECG. In this way accuracy, diagnostic quality and confidence in the ECG interpretation can be increased. For standards to be widely accepted:

- they need to be evidence-based and improve practice
- they should be written by eminent personnel in the field of electrocardiography, or by a relevant professional group
- the language used should be accessible to all staff recording ECGs
- they should have been open for a period of consultation and feedback from relevant parties before final publication
- they should be regularly reviewed and updated in the light of new clinical knowledge and technological advances
- they should be made widely available and publicised.
- Put simply recording 12-lead ECGs to an agreed standard is the only way to consistently obtain an ECG of verifiable quality.

At the clinic:

A patient presents with severe chest discomfort and feeling nauseous. Suspecting that it might be of cardiac origin an ECG is requested. In order to obtain this recording urgently no attempt is made to locate the standardised precordial electrode positions or prepare the skin. The recorded ECG shows ST elevation and a decision is made on the basis of symptoms and ECG changes to administer antithrombolytic therapy. Follow-up ECGs recorded in the cardiac unit show no evidence of ST elevation and troponin blood results are normal.

Consider the consequences of failing to follow a standardised guideline for recording the ECG.

Suggest ways in which things could have been done differently, as far as you can justify your opinions and suggestions.

Summary of key points:

- A 12-lead ECG is a graphical representation of the electrical activity generated by the myocardium on depolarisation and repolarisation. It produces characteristic waves with established duration and amplitude limits.

- There are numerous indications for recording an ECG; these range from cardiac presentations, to coexisting pathologies and epidemiological studies.

- Accuracy is limited by non-modifiable and modifiable factors, however whilst accuracy can be improved an ECG can never be 100 per cent accurate.

- Adhering to a standardised recording protocol limits modifiable inaccuracy, improves reproducibility and diagnostic quality.

Key review questions

1. Why are there few absolute contraindications to recording a 12-lead ECG?

2. A patient has an ECG recorded daily; you measure different heart rates in each of these recordings. Are there any clinical implications?

3. What is the difference between a modifiable and a non-modifiable ECG inaccuracy?

4. This chapter has discussed inter- and intra-observer variability but what might cause intra-individual ECG variability? i.e. what would cause variability in different ECGs recorded in the same individual?

References

American Heart Association, the American College of Cardiology Foundation; and the Heart Rhythm Society. (2007). 'Recommendations for the standardization and interpretation of the electrocardiogram Part I: The electrocardiogram and its technology.' *Journal of the American College of Cardiology*. **49**(10): 1128–35.

The Society for Cardiological Science and Technology and the British Cardiovascular Society (2010). 'Clinical guidelines by consensus: recording a standard 12-lead ECG an approved methodology.' Available at: http://www.scst.org.uk/resources/consensus_guideline_for_recording_a_12_lead_ecg_Rev_072010b.pdf (Accessed 6/3/12.)

Chapter 2
Electrocardiographic anatomy

By the end of this chapter you should be able to:
- understand the relevant bony anatomical knowledge required for recording an ECG
- locate thoracic topographical markers
- identify variations in anatomical structure and how these affect ECG recording
- describe the normal cardiac conduction system.

Most introductory ECG material provides an overview of the cardiac anatomy and conduction system. Whilst this is essential for interpreting ECGs its value is limited when learning how to record them. For accurate electrode placement knowledge of the anatomy of the limbs and thorax is essential. The ability to identify the bony anatomy and topographical reference lines is necessary for the correct placement of the precordial electrodes. Misplacement of electrodes has been cited as a major cause of ECG inaccuracy (Wenger & Kligfield, 1996).

Limb Anatomy

The correct position for the limb electrodes in a standard 12-lead ECG is on the limb extremities. This is just proximal to the wrist and ankle level. It does not matter which surface of the limbs is used. The region of the arm below the elbow is called the antebrachium (forearm). The two bones found here are the radius and the ulna. The radius extends from the elbow to the wrist terminating on the thumb side. The ulna runs parallel down the opposite side of the arm. The wrist itself is a complex of joints the main two being between the lunate with the radius and the scaphoid with the radius. Topographically we often incorrectly identify the small protruding bump that sticks out on the side of the ulna as the wrist bone. However this is simply the distal end of the ulna. The region is well supplied with muscles which allow movement of the wrist and lower arm. From the ECG perspective it is important to be able to identify the wrist joint complex to place the arm electrodes above the joint. The topographical location of the wrist joint is easily identifiable as the demarcation between the arm and the hand.

The region of the leg below the knee on the posterior side is commonly called the posterior crus (calf). The anterior region is commonly called the shin. The tibia bone runs from the patella or knee bone down to the medial malleolus on the inner aspect of the leg. The thinner fibula runs from the lateral condyle below the knee joint to the lateral malleolus on the outer aspect of the leg. The ankle joint complex is formed from two main joints, the subtalar joint at the heel and the true ankle joint at the anterior aspect of the lower leg joining the tibia, fibula and talus bones together. As with the wrist bone we often incorrectly identify the protruding bumps on the inner and outer aspects of the legs as the ankle bones but these are in fact the medial malleolus and lateral malleolus. The ligaments in the region are very strong and fibrous and include the Achilles tendon. Muscles of the lower leg and foot allow the foot to move up and down and the leg to move back and forwards in a kicking motion. For recording the ECG locating the true ankle joint at the front of the foot is important. The leg electrodes are placed proximal to the joint on the anterior surface of the leg or on the sides. The subtalar joint is of little importance since placing an electrode here would require the electrode and lead to be placed under the leg making it awkward for the practitioner and possibly uncomfortable for the patient.

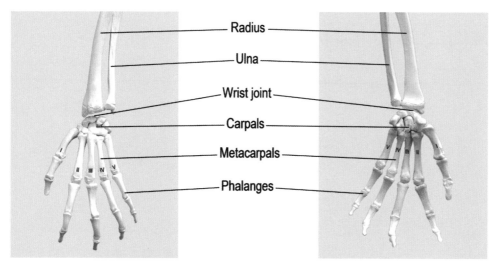

Figure 2.1: Bony anatomy of the lower arm and wrist.

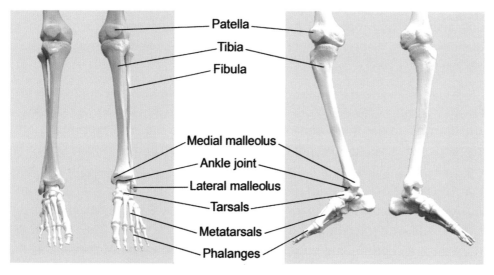

Figure 2.2: Bony anatomy of the lower leg and ankle.

Thoracic anatomy

The thorax forms the main trunk of the body and consists of a bony cage formed from the sternum, ribs, vertebrae, the muscular internal and external intercostal muscles between the ribs, the diaphragm at the inferior end of the thorax, the superior sternocleidomastoid and infrahyoid muscles. Inside the bony/muscular structure is the thoracic cavity which encloses and protects the heart and lungs, the great vessels, oesophagus and trachea. The thoracic rib cage and associated muscles are also responsible for generating the negative pressure required for inspiration.

The sternum lies to the front of the thorax running centrally down the ribcage. It is divided into three main parts. The manubrium is the upper portion joined to the first rib. Above the manubrium is the suprasternal notch, this is the large visible V shaped dip. The middle body section connects to the manubrium at a joint called the angle of Louis also known as the sternal angle or the sternomanubrial junction. This joint is sometimes visible but is easily palpable in most individuals except in the excessively muscled or morbidly obese. The angle of Louis lies approximately 5cm below the suprasternal notch and is a crucial landmark for locating several cardiac and pulmonary structures such as the aortic arch and the bifurcation of the trachea into the right and left bronchi. It is important in electrocardiography to locate the precordial electrode positions. From here the ribs and intercostal spaces below can be palpated and counted. The second rib pair is attached to the sternal body at the angle of Louis and immediately below is the second intercostal space.

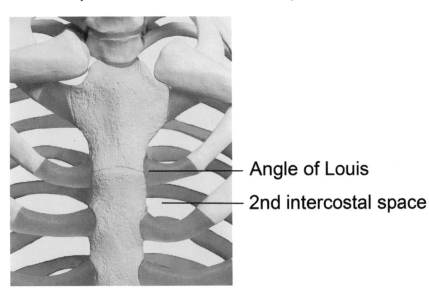

Figure 2.3: Detail of angle of Louis.

Clinical tip

When learning to identify the angle of Louis or in a patient where the angle is difficult to feel a useful tip is to use two cotton tipped swab sticks. With the patient in the supine position, lay one swab against the skin running down the manubrium and the other running down the main sternal body. The region where the two swabs cross is the angle of Louis.

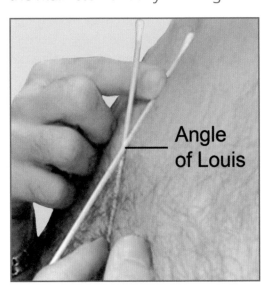

Figure 2.4: The angle of Louis swab stick method.

The rib is always felt above its corresponding intercostal space. It is recommended to count from the second intercostal space to locate the fourth and fifth intercostal spaces (SCST, 2010). When counting down the ribs the intercostal spaces should feel springy under the pad of the fingertip whilst the ribs themselves feel harder and in thinner individuals the slightly curved surface of the rib can be detected. In rare cases the angle of Louis may be located at the third intercostal space. When locating the V1 (C1) and V2 (C2) positions if they appear too low or too high it is useful to perform a double check using another method of counting the ribs and rib spaces (page 21). The distal sternum is called the xiphoid process.

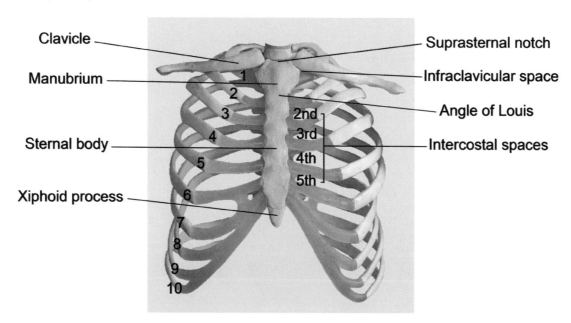

Figure 2.5: Bony anatomy of the thorax.

There are twelve sets of ribs. The first seven sets articulate with the sternum. Ribs eight to ten attach to the sternum indirectly. The remaining two ribs are known as floating ribs as only one end is attached to the spine, the other end lies free.

The intercostal spaces are also important to determine the width of the sternum for electrode placement. On average the sternal body measures 3.07cm in males and 2.71cm in females at its widest point (Selthofer *et al.* 2006). This is important for positioning the V1 and V2 where the centre of the electrode active face is placed on the sternal border. Slight differences in the sternal body breadth are accounted for by minor ethnic differences and sternal dysmorphology. As a rough check if V1 and V2 are positioned any greater than 3.5cm apart they are likely to be in the incorrect position and require rechecking. Likewise the average length of the sternum from the suprasternal notch to the bottom of the xiphoid cartilage is only 15cm to 20cm. Since the sixth intercostal space will be closest to the maximal depth of the sternum, if the V1 and V2 electrodes are placed any lower than 12–15cm from the top of the suprasternal notch it is highly likely that they are not in the fourth intercostal space.

Superior and to the right and left of the sternum lie the two clavicles which are easily seen from the body surface lying just below the skin. The clavicles run horizontally articulating with the sternum at the sternoclavicular joint. Just below the clavicles and immediately above the first rib are the left and right infraclavicular spaces. These are small indentations which can easily be mistaken as the first intercostal space if unfamiliar with thoracic anatomy. The anterior aspect of the first rib is difficult to palpate as it lies below the clavicle. Therefore if the clavicular method is used as a double check, the utmost care must be taken to correctly identify the first rib and consequently the first rib space below it.

Topographical markers

Topographically, the thorax surface can be divided by a number of imaginary reference lines. The lines on the left side of the thorax are important in the standard 12-lead ECG electrode placement and those on the right are useful when extra right-sided electrodes are indicated as for example in the case of right ventricular infarction. The left reference lines relevant to recording the ECG are the left midclavicular line, the left anterior axillary line, the left midaxillary line.

The left midclavicular line runs vertically through the midshaft of the left clavicle halfway between the shoulder and sternal ends (Rytand, 1968). This line was historically and unfortunately known as the mammary line which has led to the common misconception that the position of the nipple marks this line. The midclavicular line does not necessarily pass through the nipple when standing or lying supine particularly in females. The nipple should never be used as a guide for placing V4 (C4) underneath it. A study in 2001 by Beer *et al.* examined 100 healthy normal weight males aged 20 to 36. The nipple was located in the fourth intercostal space in 75 per cent of cases meaning electrode placement below the nipple would be on the fifth rib, and in the fifth intercostal space in 23 per cent meaning placement below the nipple would be on the sixth rib. Aging and sagging of the skin with or without obesity is likely to increase the variation in nipple position. The same study noted that there was also variation from the centre of the nipple and the midclavicular line. The closest correlation depended upon the circumference of the thorax at 2.4cm + [0.09 × circumference of thorax (cm)].

The left anterior axillary line runs vertically down from the anterior axillary fold at the front of the armpit and is the line on which the V5 (C5) electrode is placed. A common method of locating the anterior axillary line is to place the left arm by the patient's side close into the body. A fold of skin or crease is seen at the front of the armpit; this fold is then traced down the chest. This technique may be problematic as more than one skin fold can appear confronting the practitioner with a choice. The fold can also be displaced in obesity. A better method is to abduct (raise) the arm at 90 degrees to the body supporting the elbow, the elbow can be straight or bent upwards as the patient prefers for comfort. The short fold is located as the raised outline of the lateral wall of the pectoralis major muscle (see figure 2.6). The V6 (C6) electrode is placed on the left midaxillary line (figure 2.7) which runs from the centre of the left armpit vertically downwards. It is located by abducting the arm at 90 degrees to the body and locating the centre of the armpit from which the line is traced down the body.

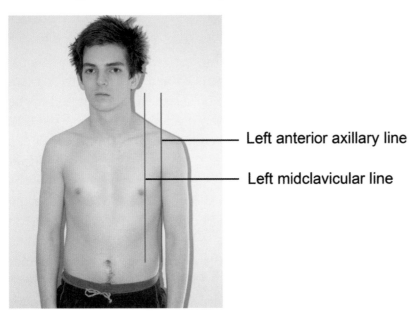

Left anterior axillary line

Left midclavicular line

Figure 2.6: Anterior thorax topographical marker lines used for locating the precordial electrode positions.

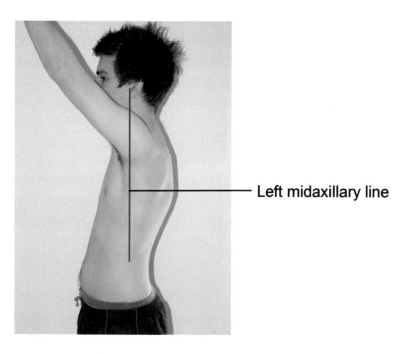

Figure 2.7: Left lateral thorax with left midaxillary line shown.

Clinical tip

- The nipples cannot be used as an anatomical marker.
- The nipples are not always located at the level of the fourth intercostal space particularly in adult females, males with developed breast tissue and in the obese.
- The nipples do not lie on the midclavicular line.
- There can be dissymmetry in nipple position on both sides of the thorax.

Anatomical and pathological abnormalities affecting ECG recording

Pectus excavatum

Pectus excavatum (funnel chest) is a congenital defect of the sternum and costal cartilage more common in males than females. The chest has a concave depression displacing the position of the heart underneath which progresses with age. Electrically the position of the heart will alter the ECG waveforms requiring careful analysis and reporting. Technically the concave depression which can be 3cm or deeper from the anterior chest wall can make precordial ECG electrode positioning difficult particularly in leads V1 and V2. There may be asymmetry of the chest so it is crucial that the ribs are correctly counted down on both sides of the chest and that no short cuts are taken. The spacing between the ribs may also be very different and the sternal margin difficult to palpate. Depending upon the severity of the pectus excavatum modifications may have to be made to the ECG recording technique. With modern solid gel tab electrodes even in the most severe cases once the sternal border has been found the electrodes can be accurately placed. Due to space limitations V1 and V2 may have to be recorded separately using the manual mode (page 78). Occasionally special pre-wired electrodes may be required if there is insufficient space to attach the ECG clip connectors to tab electrodes. Pectus excavatum was a greater problem when Welsh cup suction electrodes were used as the bulbs often touched each other so only one could be placed at a time. The ECG obtained may suggest right bundle branch block which in pectus excavatum may not be a true pathological finding.

Pectus carinatum

Pectus carinatum is a congenital abnormality of sternum and ribs. The sternum and rib cage show a convex outward curving shape caused by an overgrowth of the costal cartilages. Pectus carinatum it is more commonly seen in males and the distortion of the chest increases with age. The disease is also known as Pigeon chest as the curved thorax shape resembles that of the bird. Technically for recording the ECG the intercostal spaces may be uneven or enlarged. Therefore extreme care has to be taken when locating the precordial electrodes. In this case it is important to be confident in your technical ability to locate the rib spaces as the final electrode positions may look strange.

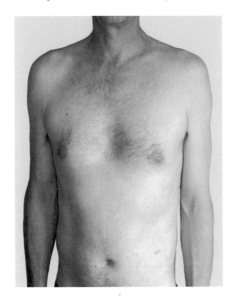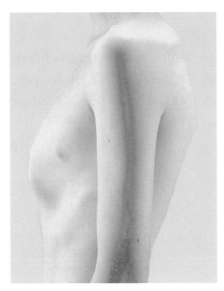

Figure 2.8: Mild pectus excavatum illustrating concave depression of thoracic cage (left) and moderate pectus carinatum with convex bulging of thoracic cage (right).

Obesity and bodybuilding

Obesity and body building would appear to be at opposite extremes in terms of body shape; however both can make it very difficult to palpate the intercostal spaces and sternum. Excess subcutaneous tissue in the case of obesity can obscure the intercostal spaces and sternal border. There is a temptation to press too hard to locate the bones causing discomfort to the patient. Additionally in obese patients there are artifactual problems due to skin stretching and movement under the electrode (page 88).

In the case of the extreme bodybuilder the development of the muscles across the chest can make palpation of the sternal edge and intercostal spaces difficult and often impossible. Unlike the obese patient pressing harder on the tissue does not afford a glimpse of the bony anatomy below. As the practitioner becomes more skilled at recording ECGs they develop a greater sensitivity in their finger pads and can detect small changes in resistance to pressure. Therefore in obesity and body building the assistance of a more experienced practitioner may be required.

Thoracic surgery/thoracic trauma

Both thoracic surgery and previous thoracic trauma can change the relationship between the bony thoracic structures. Ribs may not be symmetrically aligned or may be missing or lying at odd angles post thoracotomy. Immediately post-surgery and for a considerable time afterwards the patient's chest may be very sensitive to even the light pressure used when locating the precordial electrode positions.

Mastectomy and breast augmentation

Left sided mastectomy should not make the location of the precordial electrodes more difficult. However the presence of scar tissue and possible skin puckering may make good electrical contact between the electrode and skin difficult.

In breast augmentation electrodes should be placed in the standard locations. If augmentations are unnaturally large extending over the fifth intercostal space or are positioned over the sternal borders they may prevent the correct electrode positions being located. Studies have indicated capsular contracture and leakage of the fluid into the surrounding implant area may also make it difficult to locate the correct electrode positions accurately (Peters and McEwan, 1993).

Sharing best practice activity

Design a factsheet or PowerPoint presentation for new students or staff recording ECGs in your workplace. This should aim to pass on anatomical knowledge required for recording an ECG, and discuss some of the problems encountered in anatomical variations.

- Aim to illustrate your work with real patient cases (seek consent first and remove all identifying data).
- Get a discussion going about problems other staff have encountered.
- Organise a practical session for staff to locate their own thoracic bone structure and anatomical markers; if you have a skeleton this is useful for demonstration.

Cardiac conduction system anatomy

The region of the heart responsible for generating impulses is called the sinoatrial or SA node. It is located high up in the right atrium adjacent to the orifice of the superior vena cava. The sinoatrial node is a group of highly specialised cells which are capable of automaticity. In other words it produces spontaneous electrical potentials which in the normal individual occurs at around 60–100 times per minute. It is often referred to as the natural pacemaker of the heart. The rate at which electrical potentials are generated may change as the SA node is under the influence of the autonomic nervous system and is controlled by the cardiorespiratory centre of the medulla oblongata in the brain. The SA node is therefore affected by fear and physical activity. The sympathetic (adrenergic) division of the autonomic nervous system increases heart rate, strength of contraction, rate of automaticity (autorhythmicity) and AV conduction speed (Cohn, 2002). The heart rate is slowed by the action of the parasympathetic (cholinergic) nervous system. It decreases the rate at which the SA node fires via the vagus nerve and slows AV conduction speed. Two opposing action hormones mediate these changes – adrenaline (epinephrine) and noradrenalin (norepinephrine). Although the SA node is considered to be the pacemaker of the heart if it fails to fire any cell in the conduction pathway or in the general myocyte tissue can create an electrical potential which subsequently causes depolarisation of adjacent cells.

In normal circumstances the electrical activity spreads from the SA node down through the atria to the atrioventricular node (AV node). Anatomically the Bachmann bundle is the main route for intra-atrial conduction (Sakamoto *et al.*, 2005). Depolarisation of the atria produces the P wave in the ECG. Atrial repolarisation is too small to be seen in the 12-lead ECG but may be seen in an intracardiac ECG.

The AV node is located just above the right ventricle in the inferior-posterior portion of the intra-atrial septum. A fibrous non-conductive band of tissue lies between the atria and the ventricles preventing the electrical impulses from passing on down the heart except via the AV node and the Bundle of His (Levick, 2010). The AV node also slows down the speed at which the electrical impulses travel by around 0.1 sec. This allows time for the atria to fully empty of blood during atrial systole when the atria contract to force blood into the ventricles. This time delay is seen in the ECG as the PR interval. The delayed electrical impulses travel on down the Bundle of His which runs in the upper part of the interventricular septum. The Bundle of His divides into two fascicles or branches. The right fascicle is deeply embedded in the interventricular septum running down to the apex. It emerges at the endocardium near the base of the anterior papillary muscle and bifurcates. One branch runs along the moderator band and the other continues towards the apex over the right ventricular endocardial surface.

The left fascicle further subdivides into the anterior and posterior fascicles as the left ventricle has a greater muscle mass. The anterior portion runs towards the apex whilst the posterior travels to an area of posterior papillary muscle before both divide into the Purkinje fibres which penetrate into the ventricular myocardium. Following these electrical events the ventricles contract from the apex upwards forcing blood from the left ventricle into the aorta and from the right ventricle into the pulmonary artery. The QRS complex represents depolarisation of the septum and the ventricles. Immediately after the S wave is a period of isoelectric activity (no electrical change). This is the refractory period during which the ventricles cannot be stimulated again by further electrical potentials. The T wave of the ECG represents ventricular repolarisation. The ventricular cells return to their electrical resting state in preparation for the next depolarisation event. The conduction system of the heart is shown in figure 2.9.

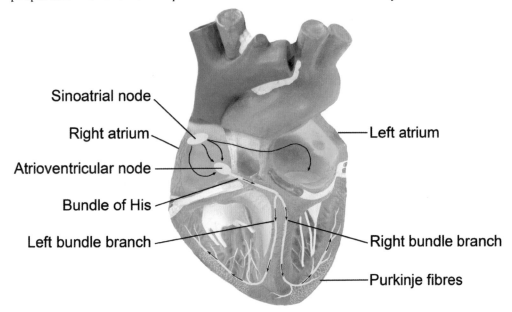

Figure 2.9: The conduction system of the heart.

Summary of key points

- Identification of the second intercostal space as a marker for locating the correct intercostal spaces is of paramount importance for recording an ECG.

- Understanding the thoracic anatomy is essential for the identification of the thoracic topographical markers used to assist the location of electrode placement.

- It is important to recognise that thoracic anatomy can differ between individuals and this may make accurate electrode placement more difficult.

• Whilst a basic understanding of the conduction system is sufficient for recording ECGs, a more comprehensive level of knowledge is required for ECG analysis.

Key review questions

1. What limits the use of the first and twelfth ribs for counting down or up the intercostal spaces?

2. Why is the angle of Louis the recommended starting point for counting the intercostal spaces?

3. You are asked to record an ECG in a patient who has undergone open heart surgery where the sternum has been split vertically to allow access to the heart. The sternum was closed by wiring. You cannot locate the angle of Louis and there appear to be extra bumps along the sternum. Why might using the swab method be problematic and what else might you try? You will need to apply your knowledge of thoracic bony anatomy to answer this.

References

Beer, G.M., Budi, S., Seifert, B., Morgenthaler, W., Infanger, M., Meyer, V.E. (2001). 'Configuration and localization of the nipple-areola complex in men.' *Plastic and Reconstructive Surgery*, **7**: 1947–52.

Cohn, J.N. (2002). 'Sympathetic nervous system in heart failure.' *Circulation* **106**(19): 2417–18.

Levick, J.R. (2010) *An Introduction to Cardiovascular Physiology*. 5th Edition. London: Hodder Arnold.

Peters, W., McEwan, P. (1993). 'Capsular contracture simulating myocardial infarction on ECG.' *Plastic and Reconstructive Surgery,* **91**(3): 529–32.

Rytand, D.A. (1968). 'The midclavicular line: where is it?' *Annals of Internal Medicine,* **69**(2): 329–30.

Sakamoto, S., Nitta, T., Ishii, Y., Miyagi, Y., Ohmori, H., Shimizu, K. (2005). 'Interatrial electrical connections: the precise location and preferential conduction.' *Journal of Cardiovascular Electrophysiology*, **16**(10): 1077–86.

Selthofer, R., Nickolic, V., Mrcela, T., Radic, R., Leksan, I., Rudez, I., Selthofer, K. (2006). 'Morphometric analysis of the sternum.' *Collegium Antropologicum*, **30**(1): 43–7.

Society of Cardiological Science and Technology and the British Cardiovascular Society. (2010). 'Clinical guidelines by consensus: Recording a standard 12-lead ECG an approved methodology.' Available at, http://www.scst.org.uk/resources/consensus_guideline_for_recording_a_12_lead_ecg_Rev_072010b.pdf (Accessed 6/3/12.)

Wenger, W., Kligfield, P. (1996). 'Variability of precordial electrode placement during routine electrocardiography.' *Journal of Electrocardiology*, **29**(3): 179–84.

Chapter 3

Positioning the patient and locating electrode positions

By the end of this chapter you should be able to:

- explain the reasoning behind using standard patient and standard electrode positions for recording 12-lead ECGs
- apply knowledge of recommended electrode locator techniques to practice
- appreciate clinical situations where standard electrode positioning cannot be achieved and how to correctly modify electrode placement in specific examples
- reflectively evaluate own practice taking into account common misinformation regarding electrode location.

Standard patient positioning for recording a 12-lead ECG

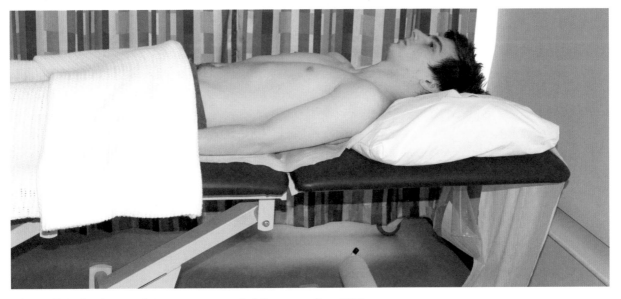

Figure 3.1: Supine position recommended for recording ECGs.

To record a standard 12-lead ECG, the patient is placed in a supine position (lying flat on back with the face upwards). The arms are relaxed comfortably by the sides and the legs extended. Limbs should be fully supported by the couch or bed so the muscles may relax. Any tension remaining in the legs may be relieved by placing a pillow under the knees. For comfort the head is supported by one standard sized pillow. Overly thick or multiple pillows raise the chest from the horizontal plane altering the spacial relationship between the heart and the chest wall. In certain circumstances, such as heart failure, the standard recording position may not be achievable. If the patient cannot lie supine for medical reasons, the head of the bed or couch may be raised so that the patient is lying in the semi-Fowler position (head raised to a maximum of 45 degrees from flat). Any change in patient position from supine must be clearly annotated on the ECG (SCST, 2010). Regardless of time or staff constraints the poor clinical practice of recording seated ECGs should not be used. Changing the patient position from supine to sitting significantly decreases ECG axis.

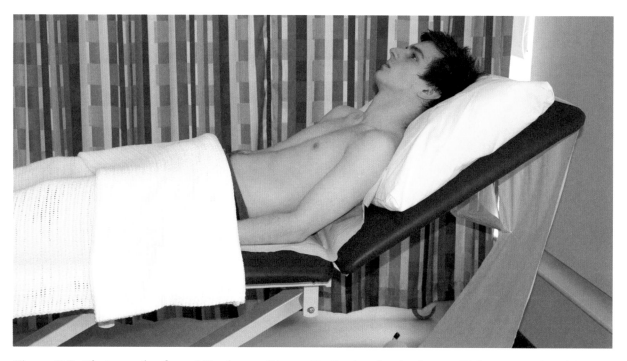

Figure 3.2: Photograph of semi-Fowler position with the head raised to a 45 degree angle. This position should only be used when clinically indicated for recording ECGs.

Standard electrode positions

Just as altering the patient position affects the ECG, using nonstandard placement of the electrodes also alters the waveform shapes and voltages recorded, resulting in significant ECG changes. Accuracy in electrode placement is required so that ECGs recorded by different personnel, in different clinical centres and in different countries can be compared with confidence. Standardisation of electrode positions does not mean that clinical practice should remain fixed in time for ever. Over the years the number of electrodes used and their positions have in fact changed so standardisation means that until a better evidence based practice comes along a patient should expect to have an ECG recorded in the same manner no matter where they are and no matter who records the ECG. This produces confidence that any changes noted represent true changes and have not been introduced by variations in technique.

Locating the limb electrode positions

Altogether there are four limb electrodes placed on the right arm, left arm, right leg and left leg. The right leg electrode acts purely as an earth connection and the voltages from the electrode are not recorded in the ECG. The standard position for placing the electrodes to record the limb leads is on the limb extremities. This is just proximal to, or above, the wrist and ankle level. The level at which the limb electrodes are placed is important with regard to accuracy and is therefore not a matter of personal preference. Moving the electrodes up the arms or legs affects the voltages and axis measured.

Before placing the electrodes ensure the patient has positioned themselves comfortably lying on their back. In terms of reducing muscle artifact it is best to let the patient's limbs remain in their natural resting position. Rotating the limbs to suit the practitioner recording the ECG may result in unnecessary muscle tension. As a result it does not matter which surface of the limbs is used i.e. the anterior, posterior or lateral surface. Although some texts recommend using the softer more pliable skin on the inner side of the arms and legs because of reduced skin impedance, this is not necessary if good skin preparation is carried out and modern low noise electrodes are used. In relation to the legs the posterior leg position is rarely used simply because it is more difficult for the operator to access, cleanse the skin and apply the electrode and lead. The patient would also have to lie on top of the electrode and lead connector which may cause discomfort and artifact.

With the patient lying in a comfortable position, palpate down either side of the legs just above the foot and locate the ankle joint (Figure 2.2). The position for the leg electrodes is just proximal to the ankle joint. Avoid the area of the medial and lateral malleolus protrusions as it is difficult to get the electrodes to stick over these bumps due to their marked dome shape. If you are unsure as to the ankle joint location, ask the patient to move their foot up and down and then relax. The ankle joint is found where the foot is capable of limited upward and good downward movement. Locate the wrist by feeling down the lower arm to the joint with the hand. Avoiding the protruding distal ulna, place the electrode just above the wrist joint. Ask the patient to bend their wrist if encountering any difficulty.

Table 3.1: Standard electrode positions on limbs for resting 12-lead ECGs.

Limb electrode	Standard position
Right arm (RA)	Right arm just proximal to the wrist
Left arm (LA)	Left arm just proximal to the wrist
Right leg (RL)	Right lower leg just proximal to the ankle
Left leg (LL)	Left lower leg just proximal to the ankle

Clinical tip

Practical help for recording limb leads
- The ankles and wrists must be exposed – socks, tights/pantyhose and stockings removed.
- Quality tracings free from artifact cannot be recorded through clothing, no matter how sheer they are.
- Remove watches or any bracelets if they affect electrode positioning.

Locating the precordial (chest) electrode positions

One of the most confusing aspects to recording a standard 12-lead ECG is where and how to locate the precordial electrode positions. Some of the confusion has arisen because conflicting information is widely available regarding placement. Scientific papers, textbooks, educational videos and tools, websites, chat rooms, ECG machine manufacturer manuals, advertising material, the press and the media all offer differing advice. The correct precordial electrode positions agreed by the American Heart Association (AHA, 2007) and the Society for Cardiological Science and Technology/British Cardiovascular Society (2010) are listed in table 3.2.

Table 3.2: Standard electrode positions on precordium for resting 12-lead ECGs.

Precordial electrode	Standard position
V1 (C1)	4th intercostal space on the right sternal border
V2 (C2)	4th intercostal space on the left sternal border
V3 (C3)	Exactly midway between V2 and V4
V4 (C4)	5th intercostal space on the left midclavicular line
V5 (C5)	Same horizontal plane as electrodes V4 and V6 on the left anterior axillary line
V6 (C6)	Same horizontal plane as electrodes V4 and V5 on the left midaxillary line

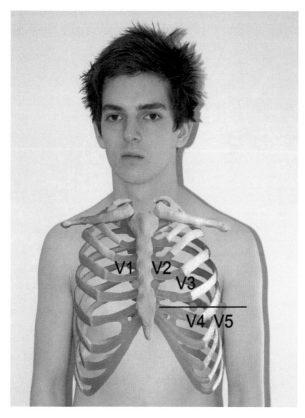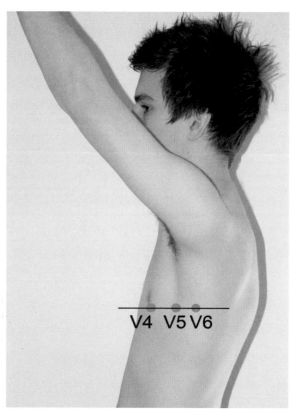

Figure 3.3: Position of standard precordial electrodes, note that V4 is in the fifth intercostal space and that V5 and V6 are on the same horizontal plane as V4.

There is a well-established technique for counting down the intercostal spaces and locating the topographical reference lines. There is therefore no place in clinical practice for the dangerous practice of 'eyeballing'. Eyeballing involves looking at the patient's chest or limbs and 'guesstimating' where the electrodes are placed. This amounts to incompetent practice.

The 'Ten Step Technique'

The ten step technique for locating the precordial electrodes has been previously described by the authors (Crawford and Doherty, 2008). There are two main techniques: the angle of Louis and the clavicular methods. The recommended method to use is the angle of Louis (SCST, 2010) and is described in ten detailed steps below.

1. Place fingers into the suprasternal notch above the top of the manubrium. Run fingers carefully down the sternum until a bony horizontal ridge is felt. This is the angle of Louis (sternal angle) formed by the joint of the manubrium to the mid sternum. As a very rough average guide the angle of Louis is 3.8cm below the suprasternal notch.

2. Keeping a finger on the angle of Louis, slide the other fingers down and slightly to the left (patient's right) until a softer more yielding region is reached. This is the second right intercostal space.

3. From here slide over the third rib into the third intercostal space and then over the fourth rib into the fourth intercostal space.

4. In the fourth intercostal space slide the tip of the finger towards the sternal edge. (Take care to press fingers inwards and not pull the skin as this contributes to inaccurate electrode placement.) Place the centre of the active face of the electrode on the sternal edge vertically and in the centre of the intercostal space horizontally. This is the correct V1 position.

5. Now repeat the process described in steps one to four above on the left side of the chest to locate the fourth left intercostal space. This is the correct V2 position. (N.B. It is poor practice to slide fingers across the sternum from V1 into what appears to be the corresponding fourth left intercostal space.)

6. Allowing for individual anatomical variation it is unlikely that the V1 and V2 electrodes would be any further apart than 3.5cm in the largest framed male. Look at the V1 and V2 positions and recheck the distance they are spaced apart is correct.

7. V4 must now be located before V3. Count down the ribs and intercostal spaces to the fifth left intercostal space. Track the path of the space towards the left side of the chest. Remember the fifth intercostal space does not lie in a straight horizontal plane to the left but moves downwards first then slightly upwards. Continue to track the fifth intercostal space until approximately the middle of the clavicle is reached. In females you must lift the breast to do this. Now keeping one finger pad in this position use your other hand to feel for the medial (sternal) end and the lateral (acromial) end of the left clavicle. Locate the midpoint between the medial and lateral clavicular ends and trace this position vertically down the chest. This is the midclavicular line. The central point at which the midclavicular line meets the fifth intercostal space is the correct position of V4.

8. V3 is now placed on the midpoint between V2 and V4.

9. To position V5, close the patient's arm against their chest. Look for the fold/crease of skin at the front of the armpit, or raise the arm above the head to identify it. Trace with finger pads vertically downward, this is the left anterior axillary line. With the other hand trace a line horizontally across from V4. The centre point where the two lines meet is the correct V5 position. Note that V5 is in the same horizontal plane as V4 but it is not in the fifth intercostal space.

10. Move the patient's arm away from the chest and locate the centre of the armpit. Trace a line vertically down the body, this is the midaxillary line. Use the other hand to trace horizontally across from V4 and V5. V6 is placed where the two lines meet.

The clavicular method is used as a double check of the precordial electrode positions. To use the clavicular method, locate the infraclavicular space indentation directly below the clavicle. Feel immediately downwards for the first rib just below this space. Slide the finger pads down over the first rib and into the first intercostal space. Place the little finger in the first intercostal space, then slide the ring finger over the second rib and into the second intercostal space. Now slide the middle finger over the third rib into the third intercostal space and finally the index finger over the fourth rib into the fourth intercostal space. From this point follow the same instructions as described in the ten steps above to locate the standard precordial electrode positions.

Locating the alternative V5 position midway between V4 and V6

When the anterior axillary line cannot be located due to poor definition a suggested alternative from the AHA (2007) is to place the V5 electrode midway between V4 and V6. The ten step method described above may be used to locate V4 and V6, using a flexible tape measure held horizontally tightly against the skin. The tape measure should pass through the horizontal centre of the active face of the V4 and V6 electrodes. Measure the distance between the vertical centres of the active face of the electrodes keeping the tape measure on the correct horizontal plane. Divide this measurement by two and locate V5 on the chest using the tape measure. Annotate on the ECG if V5 has been obtained in this way.

Clinical tip

Practical help for recording precordial leads

- The chest must be exposed fully in males and females. Do not try to locate the electrode positions by working under a bra or feeling down the front of clothing.
- Explain why you need to expose the chest, seek consent, remove unnecessary staff and family, use screens, act professionally and cover the patient as soon as possible.
- The breast should be lifted to locate the correct electrode positions
- When lifting the breast wear gloves and use the back of the hand to push the breast gently upwards. This is more acceptable to the patient than bare skin and using the fingers to hold the breast.

Problems with non-standard patient and electrode positioning

To prevent producing spurious and preventable changes in the ECG which may affect the accuracy of the clinical interpretation, the SCST (2010) warn against modifying the standard recording position and electrode location. As early as 1913, Einthoven *et al.* noted that changes in patient position cause changes in the ECG. Later studies have confirmed these findings identifying changes in axis (Jones *et al.*, 2003), a reduction in R wave amplitude and T wave changes (Gang *et al.*, 2001). Locating V1 and V2 too high reduces R wave amplitude and alters R wave progression in the precordial leads. The resulting pattern looks like the patient has experienced an anterior myocardial infarction (Zema and Kligfield, 1982). Until further studies are performed the ECG should be standardised to the supine position so that serial ECGs may be compared and interpretation is not affected. Other electrode changes produce specific ECG changes (page 107).

1. Computer generated reports

Ideally a member of the healthcare team will be skilled in reporting ECGs. It is recognised that in many environments this is not the case. Therefore it is essential to recognise that the computer algorithms used to analyse ECGs are based on criteria obtained from the supine position only. Computer generated reports in ECGs recorded from non-standard positions are therefore invalidated as any change in patient position may alter the ECG. A manual report is required which takes into account postural effects on the ECG.

2. Serial ECGs

A standardised recording position facilitates the ability to compare ECGs recorded at different points in time. Changes due to positioning may result in difficulty differentiating between true ECG findings and those that are position related.

The possible consequence of this is that clinical outcome and diagnoses may be affected (Maeder and Keller, 2007).

Necessary alteration to the standard electrode position

If there is any electrode placement deviation necessary, for example if there are burns on the chest or an open wound, then this should be noted on the tracing along with the reason why. In some centres it is the policy to leave out any electrodes that cannot be placed on the correct position, as the waveforms obtained are non-diagnostic. In others they are placed on the closest point and the new placement documented. As with altered patient position, altered electrode positions automatically compromise the accuracy of the computerised report. ECGs from non-standard electrode positions require manual reports or the computer report checked and altered as required so that these changes can be considered. To prevent later misunderstanding if altered electrode positions have been used, even if it is only one electrode, a large cross should be marked through the computerised report to prevent misdiagnosis or mismanagement of the patient.

Recordings should not be obtained from any other modified limb position unless there is a clinical reason e.g. amputee, surgical wounds, burns etc. ECGs recorded using a modified limb position must be labelled to account for changes that might affect the interpretation and clinical decisions made (SCST, 2010).

1. Limb amputation

In patients who have undergone arm or leg amputations the respective limb electrodes are placed as far distally as can be achieved. The deviation from the standard position is documented on the ECG. The limb leads should not be placed on the torso. The precordial electrodes remain on the correct anatomical positions.

2. Breast tissue

It is still currently recommended that V4 be placed under the left breast tissue in females on the correct anatomical positions (SCST, 2010; AHA, 2007). In large breasted women this may also apply to V5 and V6. In practical terms the fifth intercostal space can be just as easily located in females as in males and tracked across the chest no matter how large the breast tissue is. The only difficult part in females is that the breast tissue on occasion must be displaced upwards and held there whilst the correct anatomical electrode positions are located, the skin prepared and the electrodes and leads are applied. If the patient wants to assist in the process and support their own breast this can be easily respected. Many patients prefer to help especially when the ECG is being recorded by a male.

It has been proposed that the V4 to V6 electrodes could be placed on top of the breast. This resulted in a debate as to whether there is a significant difference in the voltage of the waveforms recorded from below or on the breast and in 1998 Rautaharju and his team examined attenuation in voltages in ECGs recorded from below the breast and on top. In the past getting suction cup electrodes to remain securely fastened to their anatomical positions once the breast was placed back down on top of them was undoubtedly challenging and often frustrating. The idea of placing the electrode on top of the breast for ease of connection and prevention of electrode dislodgement probably first arose at this time. However, suction cup electrodes are no longer recommended for clinical use due to infection risks and the majority of practitioners have moved to self-adhesive small flat electrodes with small secure connectors. The need to place electrodes on top of the breast and the need to measure potential changes between over and under the breast is no longer relevant. It simply makes more sense to continue to displace the breast, locate the exact anatomical positions and then replace the breast tissue gently back down once the electrodes are in place. The self-adhesive electrodes do not pop off and do not move position under the breast and therefore facilitate accurate and reproducible recordings of the ECG in line with practice guidelines.

It would be unlikely that an ECG recorded with an electrode above the breast would be as accurate or reproducible as breast tissue is prone to movement. When considering serial ECGs breast size does not remain fixed but fluctuates both in the short and long term. The change in breast size can be considerable in some women during the menstrual cycle. Using an above the breast placement may limit the diagnostic value of the ECG but sufficient data is not available. Using an above the breast placement may therefore limit the diagnostic value of the ECG. All practitioners who record ECGs must be capable of accurately locating the correct electrode positions.

In the UK and Ireland cardiac clinical physiologists (CCPs) and assistant CCPs are trained to record ECGs as part of their professional role. They record the largest number of ECGs and are very active in teaching other professional groups to record and interpret ECGs. It has always been their practice to accurately place the V4 to V6 electrodes under the breast on the correct anatomical positions. This adherence to guidelines has been a fundamental aspect of training since the beginnings of the profession in the late 1940s. Indeed their professional qualification examination has always required the demonstration of this knowledge both practically and theoretically prior to the qualification being awarded. It is clear that in the over or under the breast debate, at present there is insufficient reason to change current recommended recording practice.

3. Surgically enhanced breasts

A relatively recent development is the increased use of breast enhancement surgery. In some cases of large breast implants the fifth intercostal space can be partially or fully obscured as can both the sternal edges in the fourth intercostal space. As with the normal aging process artificial breasts begin to sag with time. The skin stretches leading to the point at around ten years post implant when surgery needs to be repeated to maintain lift. Unlike natural breasts where the tissue is anchored inside the body, the artificial breast is not, and the whole implant can move downwards. Sub muscular implantation can help prevent premature sag. In some individuals marked scar tissue is created under the breast which may increase with repeated replacements. Scar tissue has higher electrical impedance and does not conduct the voltages as well as unscarred skin. The effect of prosthetic breast tissue on the ECG if any has not been established. Any alterations to the recording of the ECG should be annotated on the ECG. Electrodes which cannot be located accurately can either be left out or placed as close as possible to the correct position according to local protocol.

4. Burns and skin problems

Electrodes cannot be placed on skin where its integrity has been compromised. This would include burns and skin conditions such as severe psoriasis where the skin is damaged and therefore prone to infection and stripping of the surface when the electrodes are removed. Relevant infection control methods should be employed and gloves worn for locating the electrodes. Leads on the ECG cable should be disinfected pre and post recording and as little of the leads placed in contact with the damaged skin as possible. Careful skin preparation is required, alcohol wipes dry the skin and soap and water may cause further irritation. In addition these areas are often covered in greasy medications which will cause wandering baseline artifact (page 88). In extensive burns and severe skin conditions skin preparation may not be possible at all and sub optimal tracings may have to be accepted until the skin heals.

If cardiac rhythm only needs to be determined, electrodes may be placed on the standard anatomical positions where the skin is unaffected. Where the skin is damaged some electrodes and therefore leads may have to be left out. The alternative is to reposition electrodes on intact skin as close as possible to the correct electrode positions and document this on the ECG recorded. Although very rare, if there is a major clinical reason to record an accurate ECG or serial ECGs from the correct anatomical positions regardless of skin condition, needle electrodes, surgical staples or steel sutures can be used which are connected to the ECG lead via sterilised crocodile clips.

Skin conditions such as psoriasis may cause skin dehydration and cracking due to a combination of a high epidermal cell turnover rate and allergic reaction. Affected areas as with burns should be avoided and electrodes not placed, or alternatively altered and their new positions carefully annotated on the ECG.

In females a common skin condition is sweat rashes and fungal infections under the breast collectively referred to as submammary candidiasis. This leaves the skin with an inflamed red raised rash. Care must be taken when preparing the skin and when removing the electrodes as the skin can be very fragile and may break open.

Skin tags or acrochordon are common under the breasts of females but can also be found on the general chest skin in both sexes. These are simply benign skin growths attached to the body via stalks. In some individuals they can grow quite large up to 1 cm or more in diameter. The use of solid gel tab electrodes have no affect when carefully removed from the skin and will allow the correct anatomical positions to be used. However care should be taken with electrodes with a self adhesive ring as these are tackier and can pull the skin tags off on removal. If solid gel type electrodes are not available and there are a large number of skin tags, modifications of electrode placement may be required with ECG annotation; alternatively it may not be possible to place some electrodes.

5. Neonates and babies

Locating the correct anatomical positions for the ECG electrodes in a tiny premature baby can be very difficult. The ribs are hard to feel and the intercostal spaces are very narrow. Very little pressure can be applied to the thorax when feeling for the intercostal spaces and the adult finger pad is larger than the spaces. Because of the difficulty in locating the electrode positions where serial ECGs are required the chest should be marked to keep electrode placement variation to a minimum. As well as the standard ten electrodes for a 12-lead ECG additional electrodes may be applied routinely. These include V3R, V4R and V7. V4R and V3R are located on the right hand side of the chest. V4R must be placed first and is located in the fifth intercostal space on the right midclavicular line; it is attached to the V1 lead. V3R is placed midway between V4R and V1 and is attached to the V2 lead. V7 is located on the left hand side of the chest on the same horizontal level as V4, V5 and V6 on the posterior axillary line and is attached to the V3 lead. A second ECG is recorded with V4R, V3R and V7 replacing the standard V1, V2 and V3 leads. These additional leads provide information in the case of congenital structural abnormalities.

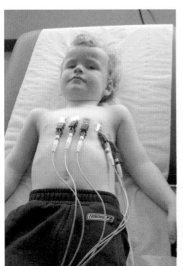 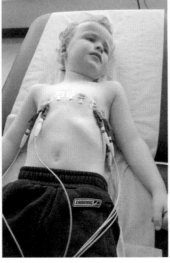 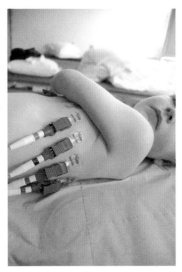

Figure 3.4: Electrode positioning in a paediatric patient.

The image on far left shows standard 12-lead ECG precordial electrode placement. The middle image shows positioning of the additional paediatric leads V4R and V3R and the far right image shows the V7 position.

6. Dextrocardia

Mirror image dextrocardia is rare but where a patient has confirmed transposition of the right and left atria and ventricles it is usual to place the chest electrodes and limb leads in completely reversed positions as described in table 3.3. It is very easy when swapping all the leads over to incorrectly attach the leads to the wrong electrodes so great care should be taken to get the new sequence right. Technically speaking there is little difference when the right and left leg leads are swapped over but to avoid confusion the whole lead set is switched. The right and left arms must definitely be swapped as the main direction of electrical potential flow will be from left to right instead of right to left as occurs in the normal heart. The ECG should be clearly annotated in regards to lead reversal and the reason stated.

Table 3.3: Electrode positions used in confirmed dextrocardia.

Electrode	Position used for dextrocardia
Right arm (RA)	Left arm just proximal to the wrist
Left arm (LA)	Right arm just proximal to the wrist
Right leg (RL)	Left lower leg just proximal to the ankle
Left leg (LL)	Right lower leg just proximal to the ankle
V1R (C1R)	4th intercostal space on the left sternal border
V2R (C2R)	4th intercostal space on the right sternal border
V3R (C3R)	Exactly midway between V1R and V4R
V4R (C4R)	5th intercostal space on the right midclavicular line
V5R(C5R)	Same horizontal plane as electrodes V4 and V6 on the right anterior axillary line
V6R(C6R)	Same horizontal plane as electrodes V4 and V5 on the right midaxillary line

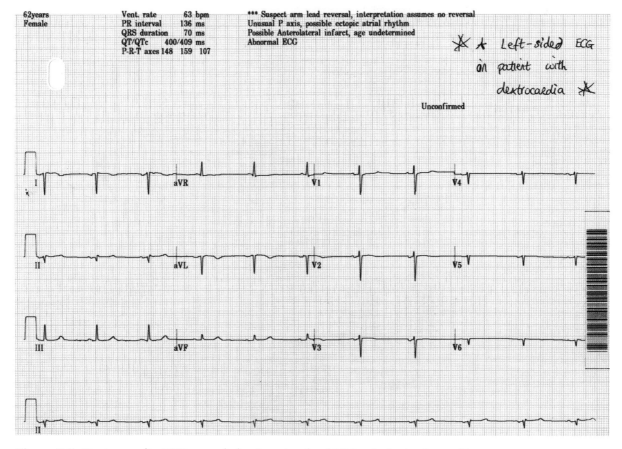

Figure 3.5: Dextrocardia ECG recorded using standard 12-lead electrode positions.

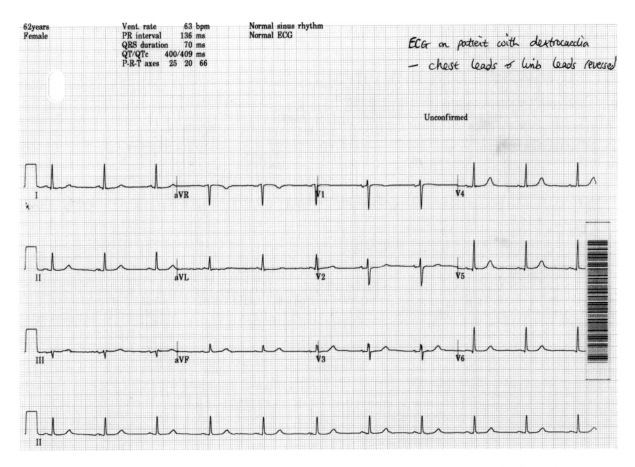

Figure 3.6: ECG recorded in the same patient with all electrodes reversed as described in table 3.3.

7. Post defibrillation

It is usual to record a full 12-lead ECG following initial stabilisation of a patient immediately after a cardiac arrest. If metal defibrillator paddles are used the skin should be very carefully cleaned of electrolyte gel to prevent slipping of electrodes and electrolyte bridging (page 99). Since the paddles are housed on the defibrillator itself and not held on the chest once defibrillation has taken place there should be no problems accessing the correct anatomical precordial electrode positions, unless there has been trauma to the chest.

On the other hand with modern and automatic defibrillators, self-adhesive defibrillator electrodes are used and are normally left in place so that the patient remains connected to the defibrillator in the initial period of recovery. Self-adhesive defibrillator electrodes typically measure 140 x 115 mm (5.5 x 4.5 inches) and are placed in one of two positions:

- Anterolateral – one defibrillator electrode is placed to the right of the upper sternum, below the clavicle, and the other is placed with the centre of the long axis of the electrode running down the left midaxillary line
- Anteroposterior – one defibrillator electrode is placed over the left side of the chest under the clavicle and the other electrode is placed on the left side of the back below the shoulder blade

Anterolateral positioning of the defibrillator paddles may interfere with locating V1, V4, V5 and V6 depending upon the size of the thorax, whilst anteroposterior positioning may interfere with locating V2, V3 and V4.

Where self-adhesive electrodes remain on the chest these should be lifted to gain access to the correct anatomical positions for recording the 12-lead ECG and when completed the defibrillator electrodes can be replaced. The alternatives are to leave out electrodes or place them as close to the correct position as possible. Neither of the alternatives are acceptable as in this acute situation leaving out an electrode will not give enough information and altering the position of the electrodes can produce artifact which suggests the existing MI has been extended or a new area of the heart has become involved (Drew and Ide, 1999).

Busting myths – common misinformation

Myth 1 'It doesn't matter where the limb electrodes are placed.'

It is easy to see why this misconception arose, two different aspects are being considered and getting confused. It doesn't matter which surface of the limbs are used because skin impedance differences can be addressed by careful skin preparation. However, the distance from the extremities is very important.

When Einthoven first recorded the limb leads the electrodes were buckets of saline into which the patient placed their hands and feet. Over time different forms of electrodes were introduced and limb positioning moved up the arms and legs in an attempt to reduce artifact and gain better skin electrode contact. However with the widespread use of self-adhesive flexible electrodes the quality of the tracing is improved in terms of reduced artifact, the electrodes stick well to the skin and do not easily slip. There is no reason why the limb electrodes should be placed anywhere other than their intended standard positions on the limb extremities (Hoffman, 2008).

Although the AHA once recommended that the limb electrodes could be placed anywhere on the arms and legs as long as it was distal to the hips and shoulders (AHA, 1975; Palhm *et al.*, 1992), this statement has been shown to be incorrect as misplacing the electrodes on the trunk or above the level of the ankles and wrists produces changes in the ECG including different voltages and axis (Garcia-Niebla *et al.*, 2009). Garcia-Niebla also noted this effect is more apparent when the left arm electrode is moved. Subsequently the AHA withdrew this statement from their guidelines and replaced it with the placements of limb electrodes at the wrists and ankles.

Myth 2 'If the arm leads are placed on the upper arms then the leg leads should be placed on the upper legs, or if the arm leads are on the shoulders then the leg leads should be placed on the abdomen to maintain accuracy.'

There is only one level at which the electrodes can be placed on the limbs to maintain accuracy. Some practitioners think that by maintaining the distance the electrodes are placed from the heart in proportion to each other the ECG will not be affected. This is not true, as soon as the arm and leg leads are moved from their standard positions on the extremities accuracy is affected. One of the worst changes in voltage and axis occurs by placing the electrodes on the shoulders and abdomen.

Myth 3 'It doesn't matter where the limb electrodes are placed up the arms and legs as long as the "quality" of the ECG is good.'

Quite what is meant by 'quality' is questionable since placing the limb electrodes anywhere other than the standard positions reduces the ECG to non-diagnostic quality immediately. This myth may have arisen due to the misconception that an artifact free ECG is a good quality ECG.

Myth 4 'The ECG machine limb leads do not stretch to the wrists and ankles so if it is designed that way it's OK to place the electrodes on the upper arms/shoulders and trunk/hips.'

All ECG machines meeting the required specifications for clinical use (page 127) have four long leads designed to reach the ankles and wrists, and six shorter leads designed to reach the chest. If ECG equipment does not have this it does not meet specifications and should not be used in the clinical setting. Limb leads may be bought in different lengths and a department should have at least one lead set that will reach exceptionally tall adult wrists and ankles. Alternatives for why the limb leads will not reach include:

- The use of paediatric leads to record from an adult. Paediatric lead sets are shorter and will not reach adult limb extremities.

- ECGs being obtained using monitoring leads via a monitoring device. Monitoring leads are shorter as they are designed to be placed on the shoulders and trunk for patient comfort, ease of movement and reduction of motion artifact. ECGs can be recorded through monitoring devices but they are primarily for the analysis of rhythm only. They are not standard 12-lead ECGs for clinical use unless the lead system allows standard placement.

- The limb leads have been incorrectly replaced with shorter chest leads.
- The limb leads have been replaced with shorter chest leads to reduce lead tangle and make them easier to handle with no regard to accuracy.

Myth 5 'V1 is located in the fourth intercostal space to the right of the sternum and V2 is located in the fourth intercostal space to the left of the sternum.'

V1 and V2 are not located to the right and left of the sternum respectively. This incorrectly permits the placing of electrodes anywhere to the right and left across the chest as long as they remain in the fourth intercostal space therefore the ECG is not standardised. There is only a vertical anatomical reference provided but no horizontal reference. To allow placement accuracy both vertical and horizontal references are needed.

V1 and V2 are placed on the right and left sternal borders respectively. This refers to the centre of the active face of the electrode (figure 5.6 page 44) being placed on the sternal edge. The sternal body at the level of the fourth intercostal space is on average 3.07cm in males and 2.71cm in females (Selthofer, 2006). If V1 and V2 are positioned any greater than 3.5cm apart they are likely to be in the incorrect position.

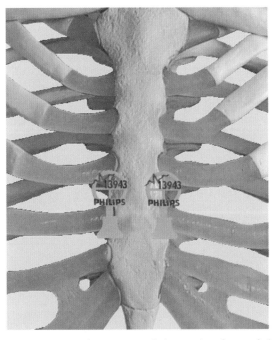

Figure 3.7: The centre of the active face of the V1 and V2 electrodes indicated by the cross hairs placed on the fourth intercostal space on the sternal border.

Myth 6 'V4, V5 and V6 are all in the fifth intercostal space.'

The SCST guidelines by consensus (2010) endorsed by the British Cardiovascular Society state that V5 and V6 should be placed in the same horizontal plane as V4 (figure 3.3). This paper is based on statements from the American Heart Association and the British Cardiac Society dating from 1938 and 1943. This means that they are in a direct horizontal line with V4; it does not place them in the fifth intercostal space. Explanatory figures of the thoracic skeleton intended to illustrate precordial electrode placement add to the confusion. Even if the correct electrode positions have been described in the text, it is common to find an accompanying figure or photograph with V4 in the fifth intercostal space and V5 and V6 in the fifth intercostal space tracking up the chest (figure 3.8).

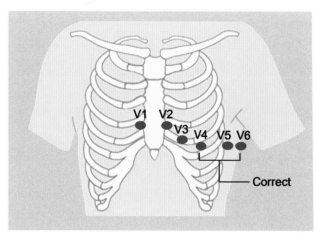
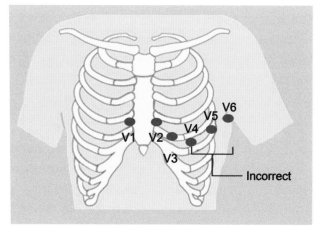

Figure 3.8: Correct positioning of V1 to V6 electrodes

The left hand figure illustrates the thoracic skeleton indicating V4, V5 and V6 placed correctly on the same horizontal plane. The figure on the right shows an incorrect diagram giving the impression that V4, V5 and V6 should be placed tracking up the chest in the fifth intercostal space.

Myth 7 'V4 sits at the same level as a bra'

V4 sits at the level of the fifth intercostal space and nowhere else. Considering the very wide range of depths available in the design of bras from standard to sports, to long line and basques etc., this statement is very misleading. The statement also suggests in some practitioner's eyes a shortcut to finding the fifth intercostal space and that the bra just needs to be pushed to apply electrodes and record an ECG.

Myth 8 'V4 is located halfway between the vertical mid-plane of the thorax and the V6 position'

V4 is on the midclavicular line. The clavicle does not run from the centre of the sternum to the middle of the armpit. Therefore V4 cannot be located by using a tape measure to measure the distance between the central sternum and the midaxillary line, then dividing in two.

Myth 9 'V5 is halfway between V4 and V6'

No. In the UK and Europe V5 is located on the anterior axillary line on the same horizontal plane as V4. The anterior axillary line does not lie halfway between V4 and V6 although it may by chance be located here in some individuals.

In the USA, the American Heart Association introduced the concept of placing V5 midway between V4 and V6 if the anterior axillary line cannot be located with confidence. The recommendations by AHA (2007) state that the V5 electrode should be placed on the anterior axillary line. Only if the anterior axillary line is ambiguous should the V5 electrode be placed midway between V4 and V6. Positioning the V5 electrode midway between V4 and V6 should be thought of as an alternative position when all else fails and the anterior axillary line cannot be located. If the midway position has to be used to record the ECG, this deviation from practice should be clearly annotated on the ECG.

The concept of using the midway point between V4 and V6 is not necessarily bad since theoretically it should increase reproducibility of electrode placement as the anterior axillary line is often difficult to determine visually in individuals particularly when they are obese. However until this becomes a standard recommendation for the recording of ECGs the current guidelines should be followed and the ECG annotated when this midway point is used.

Myth 10 'It doesn't matter if the precordial electrodes are out a bit'

Placement precision is absolutely critical to obtaining an ECG of true diagnostic quality. Incorrect positioning of the precordial electrodes during electrocardiography has long been established as a major cause of error (Hill and Goodman, 1987; Schijvenaars *et al.*, 1996; Wenger and Kligfield, 1996; Butler *et al.*, 2002). Obtaining a good quality ECG is not just about eliminating artifact. An artifact free ECG tracing is useless and may even be dangerous if the electrodes have been placed incorrectly.

The most commonly encountered problems are V1 and V2 placed too high in the third or even second intercostal space. This reduces R wave amplitude and creates poor R wave progression in the precordial leads mimicking an anterior myocardial infarction (Zema and Kligfield, 1982). Electrodes V5 and V6 are typically placed too low equating to the sixth intercostal space or lower. This alters the R wave amplitude and can falsely indicate left ventricular hypertrophy is present. Research suggests that misplacement from the standard anatomical positions by as little as 2cm can result in diagnostic errors (Herman *et al.*, 1991) and alter the computer generated report (Schijvenaars *et al.*, 1997).

One of the greatest dangers to patient care is that once the precordial electrodes are removed there is no way of telling from the resultant ECG if the electrodes were accurately positioned unless another ECG is re-recorded within a short period of time. Even then a third ECG is required to make sure which tracing is repeatable. Some changes in the ECG caused by electrode misplacement can be mistaken as true physiological changes and treated inappropriately. Whilst inaccuracy in electrode placement is not always immediately apparent an incorrectly recorded ECG is dangerous because:

- Serial ECGs cannot be compared (Drew, 2006).
- New ECG changes may be phantom artifact not true physiological/anatomical changes.
- Misplacement causes morphology changes such as ventricular tachycardia mimicking supraventricular tachycardia (Drew and Scheinman, 1995).
- Misplacement can alter the ST segment missing true ST elevations or producing phantom ST elevation (Toosi and Sochanski, 2008).
- Misplacement shifts the frontal plane QRS axis artifactually to the right (Jowett, 2004).

Summary of key points:

- Standard patient position and standard electrode positioning ensures that serial ECGs can be compared and that changes are due to altered physiology and not due to incorrect recording technique.

- The angle of Louis method is the recommended technique for locating precordial electrode positions.

- Where standard electrode positioning cannot be achieved the ECG should be clearly annotated as to the reason why and the nature of any modifications made.

- Practitioners should reflect upon their own electrode location practice and identify and address any deviations from recommended guidelines.

Key review questions

1. ECG texts frequently refer to the avoidance of bone when placing electrodes. What should you do if when locating your V5 electrode it is clear it is lying on top of a rib?

2. ECG texts also refer to the avoidance of muscle; what reason would there be for doing this?

3. Why are limb electrodes not placed on the absolute extremities i.e. at the tips of the fingers and on the toes?

4. Using your knowledge of thoracic bony anatomy, are there any other methods of locating the fourth intercostal space apart from using the angle of Louis, and the clavicular methods described in the text above or the swab stick method described in chapter 2?

References

American Heart Association and the Cardiac Society of Great Britain and Ireland Joint recommendations. (1938). 'Standardization of precordial leads.' *American Heart Journal* **15**(1): 107–8.

American Heart Association (1943). 'The standardization of electrocardiographic nomenclature.' *Journal of the American Medical Association*. **121**: 1349–51.

American Heart Association (1975). 'Recommendations for standardization of leads and of specifications for instruments in electrocardiography and vectorcardiography.' *Circulation* **52**: 11–31.

American Heart Association, the American College of Cardiology Foundation; and the Heart Rhythm Society (2007). 'Recommendations for the standardization and interpretation of the electrocardiogram Part I: The electrocardiogram and its technology.' *Journal of the American College of Cardiology*. **49**(10): 1128–35.

Butler, J., Pooviah, P.K., Joglekar, M., Hasan, M. (2002). 'Incorrectly aligned fly leads inside the ECG machine causing "ischaemic" changes.' *International Journal of Clinical Practice*. **56**(4): 298–9.

Crawford, J., Doherty, L. (2008). 'Recording a standard 12-lead ECG: Filling in gaps in knowledge.' *British Journal of Cardiac Nursing*. **3**(12): 572–7.

Drew, B.J., Scheinman, M.M, (1995). 'ECG criteria to distinguish between aberrantly conducted supraventricular tachycardia and ventricular tachycardia: practical aspects for the immediate care setting.' *Pacing and Clinical Electrophysiology*.**18**(12 Pt 1): 2194–208.

Drew, B.J., Ide, B. (1999). 'Could inaccurate lead placement cause misdiagnosis of the culprit artery in patients with acute myocardial infarction?' *Progress in Cardiovascular Nursing*. **14**(1): 33–4.

Drew, B.J. (2006) 'Pitfalls and artifacts in electrocardiography.' *Cardiology Clinics*. **24**(3): 309–15.

Einthoven, W., Fahr, G., DeWaart, A. (1913) 'Uber die Richtung und die Manifeste grosse der Potentialschwankungen im menschlichen Herzen und uber den Einfluss der Herzlage auf die Form des Eleektrokardiogramms.' *Pflugers Archiv the European Journal of Physiology* **150**: 275–315.

Gang, Y., Batchvarov, V., Hnatkova, K., Acar, B., Guo, X., Malik, M. (2001) 'T-wave morphology evaluation in healthy subjects: the effect of posture on the measurements.' *Computers in Cardiology*; **28**: 389–92.

Garcia-Niebla, J., Llontop-Garcia, P., Valle-Racero, J.I., Serra-Autonel, G., Batchvarov, V.N., Bayes De Luna, A. (2009). 'Technical mistakes during the acquisition of the electrocardiogram.' *Annals of Noninvasive Electrocardiology*. **14**(4): 389–403.

Herman, M.V., Ingram, D.A., Levy, J.A., Cook, J.R., Athans, R.J. (1991). 'Variability of electrocardiographic precordial lead placement: a method to improve accuracy and reliability.' *Clinical Cardiology*. **14**(6): 469 –76.

Hill, N.E., Goodman, J.S. (1987). 'Importance of accurate placement of precordial leads in the 12-lead electrocardiogram.' *Heart and Lung* **16**(5): 561–6.

Hoffman, I. (2008). 'Einthoven's left foot: A plea for disciplined electrode placement.' *Journal of Electrocardiology*. **41**(3): 197–201.

Jones, A.Y.M., Kam, C., Lai, K.W., Lee, H.Y., Chow, H.T., Lau, S.F., Wong, L.M., He, J. (2003). 'Changes in heart rate and R-wave amplitude with posture.' *Chinese Journal of Physiology* **46**(2): 63–9.

Jowett, N.I., Turner, A.M., Cole, A., Jones, P.A. (2005). 'Modified electrode placement must be recorded when performing 12-lead electrocardiograms.' *Postgraduate Medical Journal* **81**(952): 122–5.

Maeder, M.T., Keller, D.I. (2007). 'Sudden occurrence of Q waves: missed infarction?' *Kardiovaskuläre Medizin* **10**: 176–8.

Pahlm, O., Haisty, W.K., Edenbrandt, L., Wagner, N.B., Sevilla, D.C, Selvester, R.H., Wagner, G.S. (1992). 'Evaluation of changes in standard electrocardiographic QRS waveforms recorded from activity-compatible proximal limb lead positions.' *American Journal of Cardiology*. **69**: 253–7.

Rautaharju, P.M., Park, L., Crow, R. (1998) 'A standardized procedure for locating and documenting ECG chest electrode positions: consideration of the effect of breast tissue on ECG amplitudes in women.' *Journal of Electrocardiography* **31**(1): 17–29.

Schijvenaars, R.J., Kors, J.A., van Herpen, G., van Bemmel, J.H. (1996). 'Use of the Standard 12-lead ECG to simulate electrode displacements.' *Journal of Electrocardiology*. **29** (Suppl): 5–9.

Schijvenaars, B.J., Kors, J.A., van Herpen, G., Kornreich, F., van Bemmel, J.H. (1997). 'Effect of electrode positioning on ECG interpretation by computer.' *Journal of Electrocardiology*. **30**(3): 247–56.

Selthofer, R., Nickolic, V., Mrcela, T., Radic, R., Leksan, I., Rudez, I., Selthofer, K. (2006). 'Morphometric analysis of the sternum.' *Collegium Antropologicum,* **30**(1): 43–7.

Society of Cardiological Science and Technology and the British Cardiovascular Society. (2010). 'Clinical guidelines by consensus: Recording a standard 12-lead ECG an approved methodology.'
Available at: http://www.scst.org.uk/resources/consensus_guideline_for_recording_a_12_lead_ecg_Rev_072010b.pdf (Accessed 6/3/12)

Toosi, M.S., Sochanski, M.T. (2008). 'False ST elevation in a modified 12-lead surface electrocardiogram.' *Journal of Electrocardiology*. **41**(3): 197–201.

Wenger, W., Kligfield, P. (1996). 'Variability of precordial electrode placement during routine electrocardiography.' *Journal of Electrocardiology*. **29**(3): 179–84.

Zema, M.J., Kligfield, P. (1982). 'ECG poor R-wave progression: review and synthesis.' *Archives of Internal Medicine*. **142**(6): 1145–8.

Chapter 4
Skin Preparation

By the end of this chapter you should be able to:
- appraise the need for good skin preparation when recording ECGs
- understand the anatomy of the skin and the changes in cell structure from the basal to horny cell layers
- apply good skin preparation theory in clinical recording practice.

The skin forms the largest organ in the human body. Its main role is protection providing a physical barrier between the hostile external environment and the internal aqueous environment. The skin prevents excess loss of water from the interior, the invasion of micro-organisms and chemical assault, and provides strength, stiffness, and flexibility to resist mechanical stress on the body's surface. The skin also prevents heat loss through insulation and temperature regulation and is involved with touch and the detection of sensation. Additional functions include vitamin D production and the excretion of small amounts of waste products.

Skin impedance

Despite advances in ECG and electrode technology, good skin preparation remains necessary for recording high quality diagnostic ECGs. The skin is a poor conductor of electricity therefore when recording an ECG the practitioner encounters a phenomenon known as skin impedance. Skin impedance is simply the resistance to electrical flow. This resistance is an important source of artifact (interference) in the ECG (Davis-Smith, 2000). The higher skin impedance is, the higher the level of interference, and the poorer the diagnostic quality of the tracing. The incidence of alternating current (AC) artifact increases with higher skin–electrode impedance. Poor skin preparation also increases the incidence of motion artifact (interference caused by the skin moving or stretching).

Unfortunately even though skin impedance is responsible for many ECG artifacts the importance of good skin preparation is often overlooked. It is wrongly assumed that modern electrode design can adequately deal with the problem and so there is no need to prepare the skin. Artifact from poor skin preparation remains one of the most challenging unwanted signals to remove from the ECG tracing. As the artifactual signals are often much larger than the cardiac potentials it is difficult to electronically filter them out without affecting the true waveforms. High skin impedance arises for several reasons including the build-up of dry, dead skin cells, the build-up of dirt and grease, the use of chemicals on the skin, the presence of excess hair and as a result of psychological factors such as fear which produces sweat. The practitioner can reduce skin impedance primarily by preparing the skin under the ECG electrode sites adequately before application. Although this adds a little extra time to the recording period it frequently saves time in the long run, as electrodes do not need to be reapplied and a high quality tracing is obtained on the first attempt. To understand fully how skin impedance arises and how skin preparation controls it, it is necessary to review the anatomy of the skin.

Structure of the skin

The skin is composed of the outer epidermis, the middle dermis, and the inner hypodermis. Only the epidermis is involved in improving ECG quality through physical means. In simple terms the epidermis consists of four layers in the regions of skin used for ECG recording (figure 4.1):

- Basal cell layer (stratum basale) – this is the bottom layer where epidermal cells originate and are well hydrated. This layer has good conductivity and reduced electrical impedance.

- Squamous cell layer (stratum spinosum) – here the cells begin to flatten and move towards the surface of the skin.

- Granular cell layer (stratum granulosum) – this is the layer where epidermal cells mature, function, start to degenerate and dry out.

- Horny cell layer (stratum corneum) – this is the outer visible layer of skin consisting of cornified flat, dry and dead cells. It acts as an electrical insulator i.e. the layer has high impedance and does not conduct electricity easily.

At the clinic

A car mechanic presents for an ECG with ingrained black motor vehicle oil on his lower arms. Normal skin preparation has been completed and an ECG recorded, however on the tracing very poor signals are obtained.

What would you do in this situation regarding skin preparation?

Would you make any modification to electrode choice?

What other aspects of a car mechanic's work might cause problems in ECG quality?

Preparing the skin for electrode application

The most effective way of reducing skin impedance and improving ECG quality is to improve the electrical conduction process by carefully preparing the horny to granular cell layers of the epidermis (Farinha *et al.*, 2006). The surface of the epidermis is covered in furrows, hair follicles, sweat pores and rough loose corneocytes (hexagonal flat cells without a nucleus). Overall this provides a rough, uneven topography on which we need to achieve good contact with the active electrode face. The stratum corneum and the stratum granulosum continue to renew themselves every 6 to 30 days. Cells are shed from the outside and are continually replaced by new ones from below. The outermost cells have a reduced capacity to bind with water and have a rigid cornified cell wall, hence the increased impedance to electrical flow. Skin preparation techniques are poorly defined in the literature and vary between centres and individual practitioners. Their overall effectiveness and discomfort to the patient varies and some older techniques such as scratching the skin with a needle now conflict with infection control requirements.

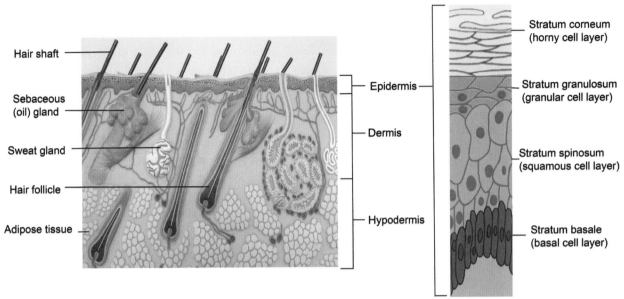

Figure 4.1: Structure of the skin.

There is insufficient evidence on how to best prepare the skin for recording an ECG. However, when combined with evidence for recording other electrical potentials from the skin surface there are a number of common features to consider. The most important factor is the light abrasion of the skin surface under the electrode sites (Farinha *et al.*, 2006). Abrasion has been shown to reduce skin impedance and artifact, and when performed lightly has little probability of skin irritation (Medina *et al.*, 1989). Light abrasion removes the loose dry portions of the horny cell layer. This may be achieved by gently rubbing with a disposable dry gauze wipe, or by using disposable ultrafine grade sandpaper (200 – 400 grit). Three to five strokes is usually sufficient at each position, however even one stroke can improve impedance. A reduction in skin impedance using a skin preparation technique which includes abrasion has been demonstrated by Oster in 2000. The other advantage of using very light abrasion is that by removing some of the oils and skin debris, electrode motion artifact may also be reduced as the electrode sticks closer to the skin.

Sandpaper designed for skin preparation may be purchased in small finger sized strips with self-adhesive backs or on a roll. Alternative less common methods of abrasion include fibrous ECG preparation pads and abrasive gels containing gritty material. After abrading, the skin should be left pink but not markedly red or visibly scratched. It takes practice to perfect this technique so extreme care should be taken to ensure not too much pressure or speed of abrasion is used. A further wipe with clean gauze or a paper towel is all that is required in most cases to remove the remaining loose cells on the skin surface. However in some cases further skin preparation will be necessary.

In hairy individuals removal of hair in the areas under the electrodes is recommended (SCST, 2010). On average the human skin contains between forty and seventy hair follicles per square cm. Therefore, the practice of trying to part and flatten the hair is ineffective since it still allows the hair to form a barrier between the electrode and the skin surface. Adhesion of the electrode is reduced and the potential for motion artifact increased. In addition electrolyte contact and penetration into the skin crevices for hydration and signal pickup is reduced if hair is not removed. The need to remove hair should be explained to the patient and consent obtained before using surgical preparation hair clippers to do this. The use of razors with blades is not recommended due to infection control and skin injury risks. Hair should be removed in the direction of growth to prevent pulling and catching. Oil and sweat is found naturally on the skin surface where it acts as a barrier to moisture loss. In patients with very oily skin or in those who have used skin lotions, it may be necessary to cleanse the skin. A mild soap solution in most cases will be sufficient to remove any oils from the skin surface. In more extreme cases an alcohol based cleanser may be required. As alcohol is highly inflammable and is also a skin irritant, care should be taken with its use. Time must be allowed for the alcohol to fully evaporate before the electrodes are applied or problems may be encountered with adhesion. Alcohol can also dry the outer layer of skin and so increase impedance in some cases. Some products also contain glycerin or oil to prevent drying but this increases electrical impedance again. For these reasons alcohol should only be used where indicated and not employed as a standard skin preparation technique. Further light abrasion may be required after alcohol cleansers have been used.

Clinical tip

Extreme care should be taken during skin preparation in patients with sensitive skin (SCST, 2010). Check suitability of cleaning products with patient before use. However a supply of the following should be readily available:

- *Bottles of sterile water and soft cleansing cloths*
- *Non greasy, soap free and hypoallergenic skin cleansers*
- *Hypoallergenic electrodes to use following skin preparation*

Excess abrasion of the skin and alcohol cleansers should be avoided.

Regardless of the final protocol chosen for skin preparation the same technique must be applied to all electrode sites as inconsistent skin preparation introduces skin impedance imbalance between electrodes resulting in increased artifact. It has been recommended that electrodes should also be allowed a short stabilization period before recording. Good skin preparation improves ECG quality by improving the electrical contact between the skin and the electrode. But the need for skin preparation may be ending. The most recent research into electrode design has been based around developing dry electrodes, and specialised coatings which use electro-optic techniques for recording which does not require electrical contact in the same way as current ECG electrodes (Fernandes *et al.*, 2010).

Warning

- Do not prep open sores, burn sites, scar tissue or areas of abnormal skin.
- If skin trauma occurs during preparation the patient should receive the appropriate medical treatment for skin abrasion.
- If skin on the right leg is not prepared as well as the other electrode sites the tracing obtained will not be optimal – all sites should be prepared equally to prevent impedance mismatch.

Summary of key points

- Good skin preparation is necessary when recording ECGs to ensure maximal contact is achieved between the electrode and skin surface, electrical impedance is reduced and artifact is minimised.

- The skin under the ECG electrode sites consists of different layers. The outermost layer of the epidermis contains dead skin cells and has the greatest impact on electrical impedance. Therefore this is the area of focus when preparing the skin to ensure a good quality ECG is obtained.

- Numerous skin preparation methods exist; currently there is no standardised approach. However, to be effective the minimum skin preparation required includes abrasion and cleansing.

Key review questions

1. Sweat can make it difficult to secure the electrodes to the skin. However if adhesion was not a problem and contact was good, what effect would the sweat have on the resulting ECG tracing?

2. In this chapter hair clippers have been recommended as the most suitable method of hair removal, razors however are still commonly used in practice. What problems may arise as a result of using a razor to remove hair?

3. ECG textbooks commonly show the epidermis of the skin having a layer called the stratum lucidum. Why is this layer immaterial to ECG recording?

References

Davis-Smith, C. (2000). 'Skin preparation to reduce ECG artifact.' *Biomed Instrum Technol.* **34**(4): 246.

Farinha, A., Kellogg, S., Dickinson, K., Davidson, T. (2006). 'Skin impedance reduction for electrophysiology measurements using ultrasonic skin permeation: initial report and comparison to current methods.' *Biomedical Instrumentation Technology.* **40**(1): 72–7.

Fernandes, M.S., Lee, K.S., Ram, R.J., Correia, J.H., Mendes, P.M. (2010). 'Flexible PDMS-based dry electrodes for electro-optic acquisition of ECG signals in wearable devices.' Engineering in Medicine and Biology Society (EMBC), Annual International Conference of the IEEE. 3503 06.

Medina, V., Clochesy, J.M., Omery, A. (1989). 'Comparison of electrode site preparation techniques.' *Heart and Lung.* **18**(5): 456–60.

Oster, C.D. (2000). 'Improving ECG trace quality'. *Biomedical Instrumentation and Technology.* **34**(3): 219–22.

The Society for Cardiological Science and Technology (SCST) and the British Cardiovascular Society (2010). 'Clinical guidelines by consensus: recording a standard 12-lead ECG an approved methodology.' Available at: http://www.scst.org.uk/resources/consensus_guideline_for_recording_a_12_lead_ecg_Rev_072010b.pdf (accessed 6/3/12).

Chapter 5

ECG Electrodes

By the end of this chapter you should be able to:
- understand that the electrode acts as a transducer
- appreciate the role of electrolytes in ECG recording
- identify the best electrode for ECG recording
- demonstrate knowledge of appropriate electrode application, removal and storage.

In order to measure and record the electrical signals generated by the heart we need to provide a link between the body surface and the electrocardiograph (ECG machine) in order to achieve a recording. Electrodes are used to provide this link by conducting the flow of electrical current produced inside the body into the measuring device. On first reflection this would seem to be a relatively simple, straightforward process. However when we examine it in a little more detail, electrodes are not just providing a means via which current is conducted, they actually need to perform a transducing function too. To understand this better we need to step back a little and consider the nature of the electrical signals produced by the heart.

The transducing function of electrodes

Inside the body electrical currents or bio potentials are carried by ions. An ion is an atom or group of atoms that have a net electrical charge due to the addition or loss of electrons. This includes for example sodium (Na^+) and calcium (Ca^{2+}) ions. As the ions move either from an area where they are in high concentration to an area where they are in low concentration or as a result of actively being pumped in or out of cells, they carry their electrical charge with them creating an ionic current. It is this ionic current created in the cardiac tissue that we want the electrodes to pick up and transfer to the electrocardiograph so we can convert this information into graphical form. Once detected by the metal electrode the electrical signals are carried by electrons instead of ions (Smith and Wace, 1995). Therefore an electrode acts as a transducer changing ionic current at the skin into an electric current. This is due to chemical reactions at the interface with the skin, electrolyte and the conductive metal electrode.

The outer layer of the epidermis is dry, dead and loose. It has high electrical impedance which means it offers a high resistance to electrical flow. However the skin itself is semi permeable to ions so in theory electrical potentials should be able to pass through it. The use of good skin preparation and electrolyte reduces the impedance problem and allows the ionic current to flow into the electrolyte from where it reacts with the metal electrode and is converted into electrical current and enters the electrode leads. Inside the electrocardiograph the electrode leads are connected to a preamplifier. The preamplifier measures the potential difference between the current flows in two different electrodes (or one electrode and the average of several others), and a measurement of voltage is obtained. Voltage cannot be measured unless two or more electrodes are used. The graphical representation of an ECG displays changes in voltage over time, voltage being the force that drives the electrons to move. Voltage is equal to current (I) multiplied by resistance (R), therefore to get the best signals the resistance to current flow must be minimised, hence the importance of using electrolyte and skin preparation.

Electrolytes

Electrodes currently in use for recording ECG signals from the surface of the body use an electrolyte. An electrolyte is simply a substance which contains free ions; this allows it to conduct electricity. Most ECG electrolytes contain high concentrations of chlorine ions (Cl^-) and sodium ions (Na^+). However highly concentrated electrolytes can irritate the skin. Alternatively hypoallergenic electrolytes are now available which improve electrical conductivity by wetting the skin.

The electrode interface

When the metal of an electrode comes into contact with an electrolyte an exchange of ions and electrons takes place. In basic terms, metallic ions from the electrode enter the electrolyte and ions from the electrolyte combine with the metal electrode at the electrolyte–electrode interface. At the skin–electrolyte interface a similar process occurs with an exchange of ions taking place between the body and the electrolyte. The overall process results in the development of a voltage at the interface between the electrode and the electrolyte. The situation at the interfaces is more complex than this and also involves resistive elements in the skin and electrodes. The important point to take away from this as a practitioner recording an ECG is that without the interaction between the ions and electrons at the skin–electrolyte and electrolyte–electrode interfaces the electrical signals could not be measured. Therefore anything which affects these interfaces affects the quality of the ECG. This includes a poor contact between the electrode and the skin surface, a poor quality or rusty metal electrode, a lack of electrolyte or even too much electrolyte causing the electrode to slip. Electrolytes improve signal quality by hydrating the skin, reducing electrical impedance and providing an environment where ionic current can flow from the skin. Electrolytes used for ECG recording may be aqueous wet gel based, cream based, liquid or solid. Liquid gels are better if skin preparation has not been good. Solid gel electrolyte requires better skin preparation but the electrolyte itself is less prone to drying out than the wet gel type. Some electrodes use an electrolyte somewhere in between a wet gel and a solid, called a gum or adhesive solid; it has a slightly tacky consistency, offers the properties of both solid and gel types and has the additional advantage that the electrolyte can also be used as the adhesive to stick the product to the skin.

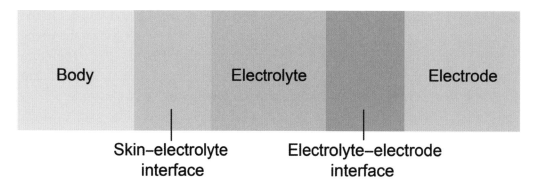

Figure 5.1: The electrolyte makes an electrical connection between the skin and the electrode at two interfaces the skin–electrolyte and the electrolyte–electrode interfaces

Electrodes available for ECG recording

Reusable electrodes

Reusable electrodes include the metal plate electrode and clamp electrode used for limbs and the Welsh suction cup electrode used primarily across the chest. Whilst these electrodes are still available to purchase, from the 1980s the culture has been to move from reusable to single use disposable medical devices to reduce cross infection risks to patients and staff. Disposable ECG electrodes are now easily affordable for all practices even when purchased in small quantities, are quicker to apply, are more likely to stay on during recording and minimise the risk of healthcare acquired infection. Studies have shown that reusable ECG electrodes become increasingly contaminated with each use, have the ability to transfer infection from the surface of the electrode onto previously uncontaminated skin, and have been implicated as a vehicle for infection (Cefai and Elliott, 1988). It is thought that bacteria are easily transmitted via reusable electrodes because of the electrolyte gel (Trend *et al.*, 1989). Whilst electrolytes are bacteriostatic, this simply means they inhibit bacterial growth and multiplication, it does not mean that the bacteria are killed. The warm moist environment keeps the bacteria alive and helps their transfer when placed on the next patient.

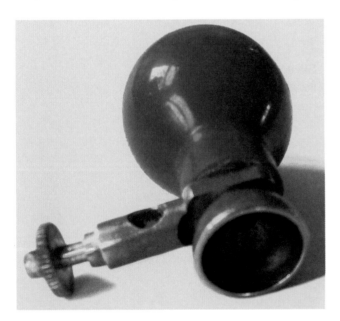

Figure 5.2: Reusable Welsh suction electrode. The electrode lead is slotted through the hole and the adjustment screw tightened to hold the lead securely in place.

Single use disposable electrodes

Disposable ECG electrodes are designed for single use only. Reusing the electrodes reduces the quality of the trace, and if reused on another individual cancels out their infection control purpose. These are the recommended electrodes to use for recording ECGs but must be used appropriately. There are two main designs in common use, the recessed floating electrode and the adhesive solid gel electrode.

1. Recessed electrodes

Recessed electrodes consist of a metal such as silver coated in silver chloride which sits recessed in the cavity of the electrode housing. The recess is filled with wet electrolyte gel, a sponge pad soaked in electrolyte gel, or a solid electrolyte gel. This type of electrode is known as floating because the electrode does not come in direct contact with the skin. Attachment of the electrode to the skin is achieved via an adhesive ring of foam or material. Recessed electrodes often use pressure sensitive glues whose adhesive property is increased when pressed against the skin.

41

2. Adhesive solid gel electrodes

This type of electrode is commonly used for ECG recording. The adhesive solid gel electrode is constructed by spreading a layer of adhesive conductive material onto a thin metallic foil backing made of silver or aluminium. The electrode adheres to the skin yet is easily and painlessly removed. They are relatively inexpensive to manufacture and have the added advantage of being thin and flexible. Solid gel electrolyte exhibits increased impedance to electrical flow compared to wet gel electrolyte. This has the effect of reducing the magnitude of the signal recorded. However, as the whole surface of the adhesive solid gel electrode is conductive and following good skin preparation, the increased impedance is compensated for. The quality of recordings made with solid gel electrodes is good.

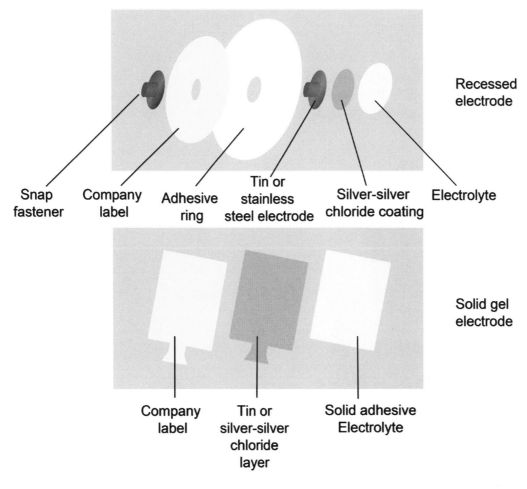

Figure 5.3: Deconstructed recessed and solid gel electrodes illustrating components.

Available connectors for ECG recording

The electrodes must connect firmly to the ECG leads to transmit the signals to be measured. There are a number of connecting devices available including snap connectors, tabs which connect to clips, and female sockets and U clips for direct use with male end of ECG lead. The choice of which connector is not crucially important when recording resting ECGs under normal clinical conditions. However if the patient is being transported, for example in a moving ambulance, offset tab type connections and female sockets with wires, produce less movement artifact. The snap connector type produces a firm secure link between the electrode and ECG lead, however if the electrode has a wet gel electrolyte it is important to connect the snap to the ECG lead before connecting to the patient to avoid displacing the gel and causing discomfort to the patient.

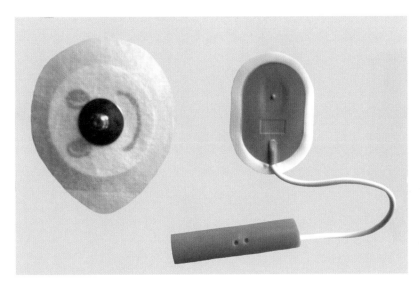

Figure 5.4: Example of a snap connector (left) and extension wire with female connector (right).

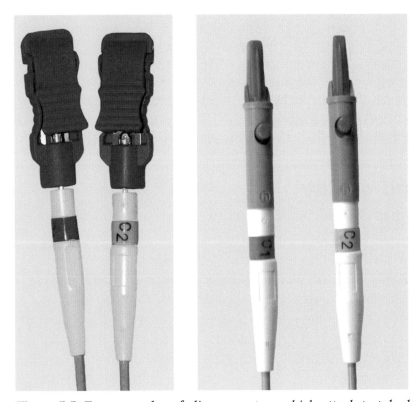

Figure 5.5: Two examples of clip connectors which attach to tab electrodes. The connector on the left also has the capability of connecting to a snap faster via a locking slit on the back of the clip.

The importance of the active electrode face in ECG recording

Not all the ECG electrode is electrically active, for instance in wet gel type electrodes the adhesive outer ring does not conduct electrical potentials. Only the area filled with the electrolyte or electrolyte soaked sponge pad can pick up and conduct the electric signal. This is important when placing the electrodes on the correct anatomical positions. The practitioner must ensure the centre of the active face is accurately placed. This may not necessarily be the centre of the electrode as viewed from above. The solid gel tab electrodes have the greatest active surface area with the whole gel area not including the connecting tab being active.

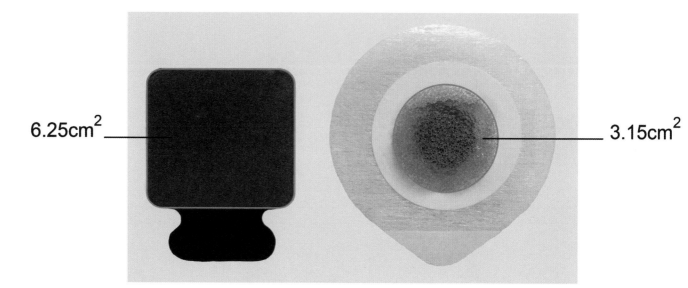

6.25cm^2 _____

_____ 3.15cm^2

Figure 5.6: Active face of tab and recessed wet gel electrode is shown inside the red outline. Anything outside of the red outline does not conduct electrical signals.

Clinical tip

When sourcing new electrodes, price should not be the main consideration. In the long run, to save money and time in relation to minimising artifact, the conductive properties of the electrode should be paramount, in particular the quality of the electrolyte used.

Electrode standards and quality

Electrodes used in the clinical setting must meet certain standards to ensure their safety and quality. These include:

- **Biocompatibility** – biocompatibility means nontoxic or injurious. In the case of an electrode it must only be used for the purpose it was intended. Biocompatibility depends upon how long the electrodes remain on the skin. For example an electrode intended to stay on for 5–10 minutes may not irritate the skin even though its electrolyte layer has a very high concentration of chloride ions. However if the same product was kept on for a longer period it may cause a skin reaction. This is one reason why an electrode intended specifically for ECG recording should not be used for long-term monitoring.

- **Electrical performance** – standards for electrical performance were laid out in 2000 by the Association for the Advancement of Medical Instrumentation (AAMI), the American National Standards Institute (ASNI) in regards to impedance and offset voltage recovery time following defibrillation. There is currently no European standard for pre-gelled ECG electrodes. When purchasing electrodes it is important to check they meet these standards.

- **Adhesive performance** – electrodes need to stick securely to the skin for the duration of their intended use. This means that an ECG electrode should be less adhesive than one used for long-term monitoring.

- **Shelf life** – the manufacturer is required to indicate the shelf life of their product within whose timeframe the electrodes, if correctly stored, are expected to remain in useable, high quality condition.

- **Reuse** – if electrodes are reusable they should have clear instructions of how they may be used, cleaned, and decontaminated without compromising the functioning of the electrode.

- **Special procedure use** – electrodes intended for use during special procedures such as X-ray and magnetic resonance imaging must have been tested for suitability in relation to these procedures.

- **Electrolyte** – the materials used in the electrolyte medium are regulated to minimise allergic and other problems.

- **Lead wires and connectors** – if the electrodes have wires as the means of connection, the wires must be designed not to fit any other devices that could result in electrocution.

Choosing the right electrode for ECG recording

The disposable, solid gel electrolyte tab design is the current electrode of choice for recording resting ECGs. When making a decision on electrode choice, samples of the different products available and their accompanying literature should always be requested from the manufacturer and a trial of the electrodes, performance evaluated. Samples should be free or supplied at a reduced rate and reputable manufacturers will always be happy to allow their product to be trialled before purchase.

There is no advantage to buying in very large bulk quantities unless you can be sure that the product will be used before the use by date. It is therefore necessary to have a good idea what current usage is and tailor ordering to demand. Remember that cheap is not always best. Electrodes should satisfy the biocompatibility and electrical properties outlined by the ASNI and AAMI, but they should also be fit for the specific purpose and department for which they are intended.

You may need to give consideration to a gentle adhesive if you work primarily with an elderly or paediatric population. On the other hand staff may prefer electrodes that are supplied in sets of 10 on a single backing card for ease of use, whilst others may prefer electrodes with individual backing. Staff may prefer one connection method over another. Departments who train junior staff may wish to consider a supply of electrodes that incorporate cross hair positioning guidance into their design to improve electrode positioning. Such electrodes are also useful to assess ongoing continuing personal development, for practical assessments and for audit of electrode positioning purposes. Above all the tracing obtained from the electrodes should be high quality when skin has been properly prepared, electrodes are correctly applied and all sources of artifact have been eliminated.

An ideal electrode is one which :

- is highly conductive
- gives rise to low stable potentials
- has low interface impedance
- has low polarising properties
- does not produce irritation to skin e.g. nickel that is not plated with another metal would not be suitable
- adheres to the skin well but is easy to remove after the procedure
- is of suitable size
- meets infection control requirements
- is pliable enough to closely fit the skin contours.

Table 5.1: Instructions for applying and removing electrodes.

Applying and removing electrodes			
	Recessed wet gel	**Recessed solid gel**	**Solid gel**
Prepare for use	Attach ECG lead if electrode has a central snap connector. Peel off protective backing disc	Attach ECG lead if electrode has a central snap connector. Peel off protective backing disc	Peel off protective backing sheet
Electrolyte check	Check gel appears wet Check within use by date	Check within use by date	Check within use by date
Application	Place on skin, run finger tips around the adhesive ring only – do not press the central gel filled region	Press whole surface of electrode firmly against skin	Press whole surface of electrode firmly against skin
Removal	Follow manufacturer's instructions. Carefully peel away holding skin around the electrode firmly to minimise skin pulling and pain. Electrode may pull out any remaining hairs. Wipe away any residue of gel left on the skin as it may cause irritation if left on	Follow manufacturer's instructions. Carefully peel away holding skin around the electrode firmly to minimise skin pulling and pain. Electrode may pull out any remaining hairs. No residue from gel should be left	Follow manufacturer's instructions. Carefully peel away, should not be painful as adhesive is less aggressive. Support the skin and pull electrode back on itself. No residue should be left. If very warm or left on skin for long time gel may become tacky. Remove residue with a tissue

Clinical Tip

Regardless of electrode design, electrolyte does not respond well to tights (pantyhose) no matter how sheer, and so should not be applied over them.

Electrodes should not be applied to broken skin, burns or recent scar tissue.

When applying electrodes place on the chest and arms with connections facing downwards, and on the legs with connections facing upwards. This allows for faster connection to the ECG leads and prevents tugging of the leads on the electrodes.

When using clip connectors ensure the metal of the connector makes contact with the metal of the electrode or a signal will not be obtained.

Some reddening and even itchiness can occur due to the mechanical stress of pulling the sticky electrode off the skin and hair follicles known as skin stripping. Carefully following manufacturer's removal instructions should avoid this. Simple reddening requires no intervention and should resolve quickly.

Storage of electrodes

Most ECG electrodes have a shelf life of around 24 months if unopened, however once the storage package is opened shelf life lasts for approximately 30 days. Check individual electrodes for specific dates. Electrodes are typically supplied in sealed packets of approximately 25 or individual sets of 10 depending on brand and design. It is crucial that the electrolyte is not allowed to dry out or the adhesive to lose its tacky property. Dry electrolyte causes electrical interference and an unstable baseline in the tracing; sometimes a tracing cannot be obtained at all as the signals are prevented from passing from the skin's surface into the ECG equipment. For this reason the packaging materials are foil lined to keep moisture in. Once the package is opened evaporation of the aqueous portion of the electrolyte can occur. It is important to maintain the viability of the remaining electrodes by correctly sealing the storage package after use. When opening a package for the first time, carefully cut or tear off as little as possible of the package at the top edge to allow access to the electrodes inside. To reseal, shake the remaining electrodes down to the bottom of the packet, carefully expel any air inside the packet and fold over the cut end twice. Hold the package edge closed with paper clips or a paper clamp. If you do not intend to use the electrodes again for several days, carefully seal the package shut with sticky tape. Consider writing the time and date a pack of electrodes is first opened to help keep track of electrode quality. The practice of removing ECG electrodes to place in a drawer or other storage area is not recommended as once removed from the bag the electrodes are exposed to the drying effects of the environment.

Since ECG electrodes have a finite shelf life care should be taken to use the electrodes before the use by date is reached and to rotate stock to use the oldest electrodes first. Because of evaporation loss from the electrolyte, electrodes should be stored in a cool area away from sources of heat.

Summary of key points

- ECG electrodes act as transducers converting ionic potentials into electrical currents that can be recorded.

- An electrolyte is a substance which contains free ions allowing it to conduct electricity. In the ECG it helps reduce impedance and increase the quality of the tracing obtained.

- There are numerous electrode manufacturers, each developing a range of products. Healthcare practitioners should evaluate a range of these before purchasing a supply for service needs.

- Electrode performance can be affected by inappropriate storage and/or application.

- Electrodes must be removed carefully following manufacturer's instructions to avoid skin irritation and damage.

Key review questions

1. What should be considered in relation to the size of the electrodes used for recording ECGs?

2. An elderly female attends for an ECG. Her skin is prepared following departmental skin preparation guidelines. Wet electrolyte gel electrodes are applied and a good quality ECG is recorded. The electrodes are carefully removed and the area under the electrodes wiped clean of the residue from the electrolyte gel. The patient is allowed to dress again and leave the department. The patient returns fifteen minutes later complaining of itchy skin across her chest. On examination there are angry red welts where the six chest electrodes have been placed. What should you do?

3. When recording paediatric ECGs is it OK to use adult electrodes?

4. What are the ideal properties of an ECG electrolyte?

References

American National Standards Institute (ANSI) and Association for the Advancement of Medical Instrumentation (AAMI) (2000) EC12-2000, R2010. 'Disposable ECG Electrodes.' Association for the Advancement of Medical Instrumentation. Arlington, Virginia.

Cefai, C., Elliott, T.S. (1988) 'Reusable ECG electrodes a vehicle for cross infection?' *Journal of Hospital Infection.* **12**(1): 65–7.

Smith, D.C., Wace, J.R. (1995). 'Surface electrodes for physiological measurement and stimulation.' *European Journal of Anaesthesiology* . **12**(5): 451–69.

Trend, V., Hale, A.D., Elliott, T.S. (1989). 'Are ECG Welsh cup electrodes effectively cleaned?' *Journal of Hospital Infection.* **14**(4): 325–31.

Chapter 6

Understanding the lead system and colour codes used for ECG recording

By the end of this chapter you should be able to:

- differentiate between the functions of the various components of an ECG patient cable
- demonstrate understanding of how the 12 leads in a standard ECG are derived
- employ the correct colour code system when recording ECGs
- relate lead orientation to underlying cardiac anatomy
- evaluate methods of displaying the 12-lead ECG tracing.

Components of an ECG patient cable

The patient cable is composed of the ECG leads, a yoke and the device end connector which joins into the acquisition end of the electrocardiograph. Designs of each piece of the patient cable differ depending upon the particular brand and model of the electrocardiograph. It is also possible to have custom made ECG cables manufactured for specific needs.

The device end connector

Typically device end connectors consist of a male pin type connector e.g. a fifteen or twenty-one pin connector. This fits snugly into the corresponding female connector at the electrocardiograph end.

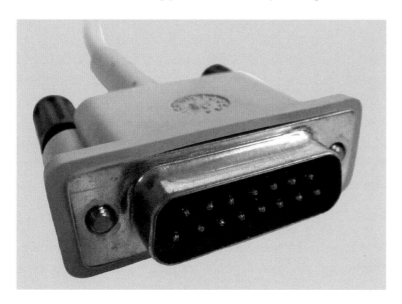

Figure 6.1: A fifteen pin ECG patient cable connector.

The cable

The cable is responsible for conducting the electrical signals from the ECG leads to the electrocardiograph. The cable is covered in an outer jacket which must meet specifications for biocompatibility and cytotoxicity as it often rests on the patient's skin during an ECG recording. Typical jacket materials include polyurethane and Santoprene™ (a mixture of rubber and polypropylene). Whichever material is used it must be flexible enough to bend but hard enough to protect the electric cables inside and be latex free. Cables vary in length depending on the manufacturer and product but are typically around three metres long for adults.

Cable components

1. Braided and spiral shields

Just under the cable jacket lies a layer of braided shielding or spiral shielding which is grounded to earth and acts as a shield against external electrical interference or noise. This includes triboelectric noise which is caused by vibration or rubbing of the materials inside the cable. As with the cable jacket the braided shield must allow flexibility of the cable. Spiral shielding is not as robust as the braided type. Over time bending of the cable can result in the shielding separating resulting in a breakdown of the shielding properties.

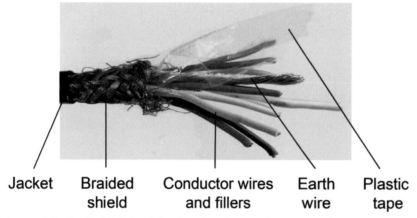

| Jacket | Braided shield | Conductor wires and fillers | Earth wire | Plastic tape |

Figure 6.2: Typical ECG cable showing internal construction.

2. Conductor wires

The conducting wires conduct the electrical signal from the electrode to the electrocardiograph for signal processing and graphical representation. Typically conducting wires are made of copper as this has high conductive properties. The trade-off is that copper is relatively soft and easily damaged if twisted so other alloys can be used instead if this is a problem. The conductors used in medical equipment are stranded rather than solid, the higher the number of strands the greater the diameter and cost of the conductor but the greater the flexibility of the cable.

3. Fillers

Several fillers will be incorporated into the cable design; these help stop movement and therefore triboelectric noise inside the cable. Fillers are simply strands of cotton or plastic which run the length of the cable.

4. Tapes

Tape is used to bind the contents of the cable together to hold them in position and stop movement. Typically the tapes are made of Teflon or plastic and are bound spirally round the cable components. The tighter the bind around the cable components, the stiffer the resultant cable. A balance needs to be obtained between functionality and flexibility.

5. The yoke

The yoke is the link between the ten ECG leads and the main patient cable. Yokes ensure secure connection between the ECG leads and the electronic circuitry including resistors for defibrillation protection and recovery. In some products individual leads can be replaced in the yoke if a fault develops without having to change the complete patient cable system. However sealed systems which permanently connect the yoke and leads are gaining popularity. In addition they prevent the possibility of connecting the wrong leads into the yoke, and eliminate loose connections. Depending on yoke design all ten ECG leads may be located along the top, called a unidirectional design. Alternatively the arrangement can be eight leads along the top with the two outermost being the arm leads and two leg leads emerging from the bottom of the yoke. This is called an anatomical design and some practitioners find this easier to use. This arrangement is thought to speed up lead connection and reduce lead juxtaposition. The yoke is frequently colour coded to match the ECG leads in either the International Electrotechnical Commission (IEC) or American Heart Association (AHA) colour code protocols (table 6.4, page 61). Yokes should be lightweight as they are typically rested on the patient's abdomen during recording.

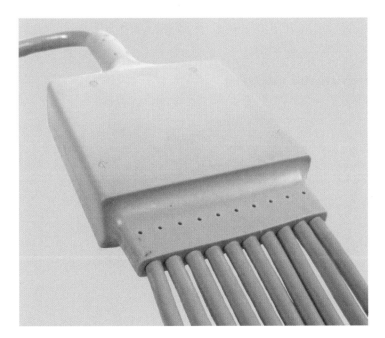

Figure 6.3: An example of a unidirectional sealed ECG cable yoke.

6. Patient leads and connectors

The ECG patient cable has ten colour coded patient leads connected through the yoke. Four are the long limb leads and six shorter chest leads. There are various ways of connecting the leads to the corresponding electrodes. Some leads have integral moulded connectors; others have 4mm banana plugs which fit into the connector. The various connectors include female stud/snap fasteners, crocodile clips and crab claw grips. Typical ECG lead length is approximately 60–75cm for resting adult ECGs.

7. Additional features

Additional features may include flexible reliefs to allow bending at the points of stress such as at the bottom of the yoke where it joins the main cable and at the cable end where it joins into the electrocardiograph. The flexible reliefs allow motion in the cable and reduce breakages of the connectors and internal wires thereby extending product life. The complete patient cable system should withstand cleaning with a damp soapy cloth and also where required cleaning with standard seventy percent alcohol solution without damage to the outer coatings.

8. New developments in patient cable design

The patient cable system is one of the most unwieldy parts of the electrocardiograph. The cables and leads frequently become tangled with use and considerable time is spent eliminating this problem. The cable and leads are also a potential source of ECG artifact. Artifact is created by breaks in the cable or shielding and cable movement. Unwanted currents can be induced by knotting, tangling and overlapping of the cable and leads (page 93). ECG leads have also been implicated as a reservoir for infection (Albert *et al.*, 2010; Jancin, 2004). New wireless systems are just beginning to come on the market where the ECG signals are sent directly to the electrocardiograph and on for processing bypassing the need for an ECG patient cable.

Derivation of the lead system for resting 12-lead ECGs

The term ECG lead in electrocardiography has two meanings. One meaning refers to the ECG hardware itself so the ECG lead is the wire connection between the electrode and the electrocardiograph. The other is the tracing or view of the heart as recorded in the ECG. So we might say, 'there is ST elevation in leads II, III and aVF'. The standard 12-lead ECG means twelve different tracings of the heart are obtained by using only ten electrodes. Nine electrodes measure the electrical potentials whilst the tenth is an earth. The 12 tracing leads are shown in table 6.1. the method by which 12 tracings are derived (or obtained) using only 9 electrodes is explained below.

Table 6.1: Standard leads used for electrocardiographic recording.

Limb leads	Precordial leads
Lead I	Lead V1
Lead II	Lead V2
Lead III	Lead V3
Lead aVR	Lead V4
Lead aVL	Lead V5
Lead aVF	Lead V6

The limb leads

There are six limb leads I, II, III, aVR, aVL and aVF. The limb leads view the heart from the frontal plane and are used to calculate the mean QRS and P wave axis.

Anatomically an imaginary vertical line divides the body into two aspects, the anterior (front) and posterior (back). When a standing person is viewed from the anterior position you are looking at the frontal plane.

The standard limb leads (Einthoven's leads)

Leads I, II and III are the oldest ECG leads recorded and are attributed to Willem Einthoven, the father of modern electrocardiography. These three leads are bipolar which simply means that the measurements made are of potential differences between two electrodes, one of positive polarity and one of negative polarity placed on the body. When recording an ECG, every electrode has an agreed upon polarity. Einthoven decided upon the polarity of these three leads so that all the tracings obtained would produce positive (upright) waves. The right arm is always negative, the left leg is always positive and the left arm varies depending on whether lead I or lead III is being recorded. The main direction of depolarisation of the heart, responsible for the electrical activity, moves from the upper right atrium to the larger lower left ventricle. As a result each lead records a different view of cardiac depolarisation. It is in this way that the ECG can be used to provide information regarding structure and function.

Lead I

Lead I measures the potential difference between the negative right arm and the positive left arm. Lead I 'looks' at the left lateral side towards the left atrium and left ventricle. Lead I is said to lie at zero axis to the heart, in other words it measures potentials or vectors travelling horizontally across the heart from right to left. A vector has both size or magnitude (measured in millivolts) and direction (moves towards or away from a specific electrode). In this case net movement is from the right arm towards the left arm.

As lead I measures the potential difference between the right arm and the left arm this can be expressed as: Lead I $= E_L - E_R$ where E_L is the electrical potential at the left arm and E_R is the electrical potential at the right arm.

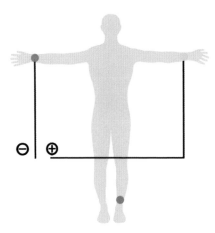

Figure 6.4: Derivation of lead I.

Lead II

Lead II measures the potential difference between the negative right arm and the positive left leg. Lead II 'looks' at the inferior (bottom) side of the heart towards the left and right ventricles from the apex of the heart. The electrical current flow or vector from the right arm to the left leg most closely resembles the movement of the cardiac potentials down the normal conduction system. Lead II is the most commonly used lead for monitoring as the P wave and QRS complexes are prominent in this lead. Lead II is said to lie at +60 degrees in relation to the heart. Therefore a depolarisation wave travelling at +60 degrees towards the left leg will produce the greatest deflection of all.

As lead II measures the potential difference between the right arm and the left leg this can be expressed as: Lead II $= E_F - E_R$ where E_F is the electrical potential at the left leg or foot and E_R is the electrical potential at the right arm.

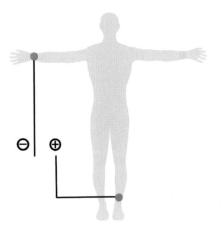

Figure 6.5: Derivation of lead II.

Lead III

Lead III measures the potential difference between the negative left arm and the positive left leg. Lead III 'looks' at the heart from the inferior side towards the right and left ventricles. Lead III is said to lie at $+120$ degrees relative to the heart. As most vectors do not travel from left to right in the heart lead III will always be small. As lead III measures the potential difference between the left arm and the left leg this can be expressed as: Lead III $= E_F - E_L$ where E_F is the electrical potential at the left leg or foot and E_L is the electrical potential at the left arm.

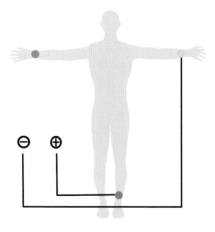

Figure 6.6: Derivation of lead III.

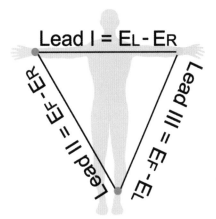

Figure 6.7: The Einthoven standard limb leads I, II and III with derivation equations.

Clinical tip

It can be difficult to remember the potential difference that each of the Einthoven limb leads represents. A useful aide memoire is:

Lead I   right arm to **L**eft arm (contains I 'L')

Lead II   right arm to **L**eft **L**eg (contains II 'Ls')

Lead III   **L**eft arm to **L**eft **L**eg (contains III 'Ls')

The tracings obtained from the three standard limb leads are similar in that when there is no conduction system abnormality, they usually all register positive P and T waves. The QRS complex is predominantly positive too although there will be small negative deflections as well. Overall the limb leads I, II and III provide little detailed information about the underlying cardiac structures but are most useful in determining the main direction of electrical impulse movement or cardiac axis.

Einthoven's triangle and Einthoven's law

The three limb leads I, II and III form an imaginary equilateral triangle with the heart in the centre. This triangle is called the Einthoven triangle named for Willem Einthoven. When we think of the average body it is hard to see how the electrodes placed on the wrists and ankles could form a triangle with sides of equal length. What must be remembered is the triangle was used to describe a concept only. This concept states at any instant in the cardiac cycle when all three leads are added they equal zero. The equation can be written as:

Lead I + Lead II + Lead III = 0

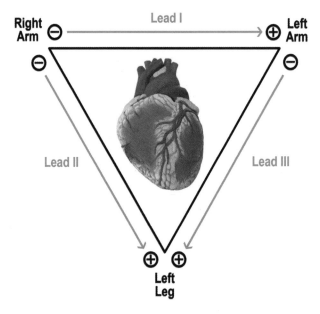

Figure 6.8: Einthoven's triangle.

However we also need to remember that Einthoven wanted his standard limb leads to be displayed predominantly upright. To do this he changed the polarity of left arm in lead II. As a result the equation must be rewritten as:

Lead I + (- Lead II) + Lead III = 0

This is more commonly written as Einthoven's law:

Lead I + Lead III = Lead II

Einthoven's law only holds true if the electrodes are placed more than 10cm from the centre of the heart. This has been interpreted as the electrodes can be placed anywhere on the limbs as long as they are more than 10cm from the centre of the heart. Unfortunately this is not true and has resulted in numerous inaccurate ECG recordings being made. This concept only refers to Einthoven's law.

At the clinic

A 50-year-old male arrived at casualty complaining of chest pain. His GP recorded the ECG shown in (a). The computerised report suggested an inferior infarction, so he was admitted and ECG (b) recorded. During recording the man wanted to know why electrodes were placed on his limbs when his torso had been used previously.

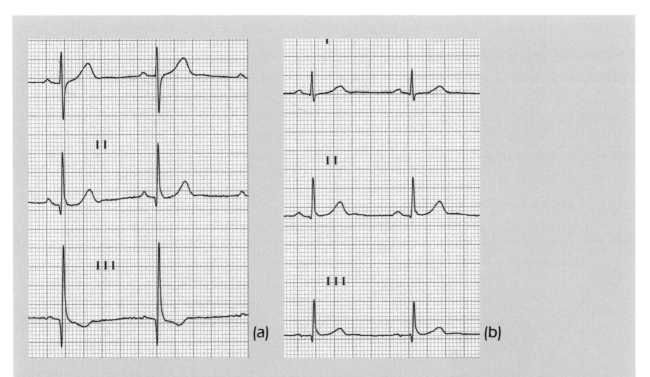

Placing the electrodes on the torso is common practice in some centres as the ECG is quicker to obtain. However it is clear to see that this has resulted in very different ECG morphology even though Einthoven's law still holds true. In figure (a) the electrodes have been moved to the tops of the limbs; the voltages now measured are lead I = -2 mV, lead II = 11 mV and lead III = 14mV using Einthoven's Law -2 + 14 = 12mV. In figure (b) the net voltage measured at the wrists and ankles in lead I = 4 mV, lead II = 11 mV and lead III = 7m V using Einthoven's Law 4 + 7 = 11mV.

Recording the ECG with the limb electrodes placed on the torso may have obtained a quick tracing at the time but what are the overall costs of this action in terms of:

- Monetary costs?
- Patient costs?
- Time costs?

What is the best way of preventing this happening in the future?

Warning

Moving limb electrodes from their standard positions just proximal to the wrist and ankle joints alters the recorded voltages and can result in misdiagnosis.

The augmented limb leads

To increase the sensitivity of the ECG an additional set of electrical perspectives or 'views' of the heart were added to leads I, II and III giving the full complement of six limb leads. Originally these were obtained by measuring the potential difference between a single exploratory (or active) electrode placed on the right arm, left arm or left leg and Wilson's central terminal (Wilson *et al.*, 1932). Wilson's central terminal (WCT) is an averaged indifferent (or reference) point achieved by connecting all limb leads together through resistors and dividing by three:

Wilson's central terminal (WCT) = 1/3 (E_R + E_L + E_F)

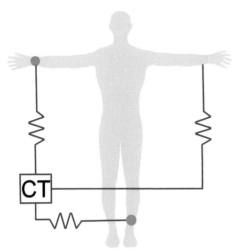

Figure 6.9: Wilson's central terminal.

Although these leads are often referred to as being unipolar they are in fact still bipolar as they measure potential differences between two points. Using Wilson's central terminal produced very thick lined and small amplitude tracings (Wilson *et al.*, 1934). The waves obtained using Wilson's central terminal VR, VL and VF were small in amplitude because the exploratory electrode potential formed part of the central terminal (figure 6.9).

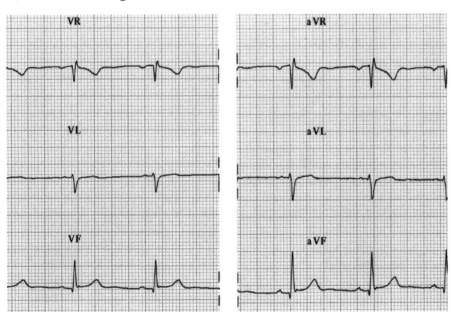

Figure 6.10: Leads VR, VL and VF are shown on the left hand side and the augmented leads on the right hand side. Both are recorded using standard calibration settings.

To increase the usefulness of these leads Emanuel Goldberger worked to adapt Wilson's central terminal by replacing the three resistors in its design with three ordinary electrical wires. Also instead of averaging the signals from all three limb electrodes, Goldberger disconnected the electrode he wanted to measure from his central terminal and simply averaged the remaining two. In other words when he wanted to measure VR he noted the potential difference between the right arm electrode disconnected from the central terminal and the left arm electrode plus the left leg electrode divided by two (figure 6.11). This process occurs inside the ECG machine.

The voltage of Goldberger's central terminal varies depending on the combination of limb electrodes used. The resulting tracings have the same morphology as the tracings obtained using Wilson's central terminal. Goldberger's central terminal augmented or amplified the tracings. Therefore a small 'a' was added to their name to indicate this. Goldberger's terminal augments the voltage signals by around 50% which makes them roughly similar in size to the bipolar leads so that they may be more easily seen and measured (Goldberger, 1942 a and b).

aVR = E_R [positive pole] − ½ (E_L + E_F) [negative pole]

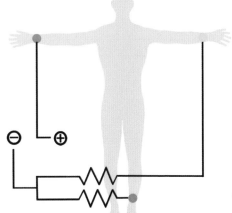

Figure 6.11: Derivation of lead aVR.

aVL = E_L [positive pole] − ½ (E_R + E_F) [negative pole]

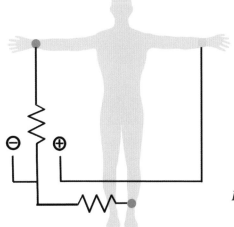

Figure 6.12: Derivation of lead aVL.

aVF = E_F [positive pole] − ½ (E_R + E_L) [negative pole]

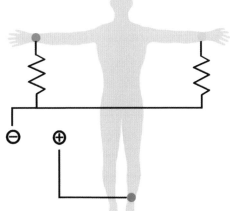

Figure 6.13: Derivation of lead aVF.

where:

E_R = right arm electrode

E_L = Left arm electrode

E_F = Left leg electrode

Lead aVR

or *lead augmented vector right arm* 'looks' at the heart from the right shoulder towards the left atrium. Lead aVR is said to lie at -150 degrees relative to the heart. This lead provides little diagnostic information as the direction of electrical depolarisation is away and downwards from it.

Lead aVL

or *lead augmented vector left arm* 'looks' at the heart from the left shoulder towards the left ventricle. Lead aVL is said to lie at -30 degrees relative to the heart.

Lead aVF

or *lead augmented vector left foot* 'looks' at the heart from the left foot towards the inferior surface of the left ventricle. Lead aVF is said to lie at +90 degrees relative to the heart.

When there is no conduction system abnormality the tracings obtained from the three augmented limb leads register positive or upright P and T waves in aVL and aVF. These leads also have a predominantly positive QRS complex. Lead aVR on the other hand is predominantly negative or inverted. This is because it looks towards the heart from the right shoulder where the electrical flow is primarily away from the electrode. The fact that aVR is negative can act as a quick check to see the limb leads have been connected to the correct electrodes. If aVR is positive limb lead reversal of the arm leads has most likely occurred (table 9.9, page 103). If the leads and electrodes are correctly placed then consider dextrocardia. Overall as with the bipolar limb leads I, II and III, the augmented leads provide little specific information about underlying cardiac structure, their main use is again in the calculation of cardiac axis.

The precordial chest leads

There are six electrodes attached to the chest in the standard 12-lead ECG. The routine use of precordial leads was introduced in the 1930s by Wilson. As with the augmented leads the precordial leads are frequently referred to as being unipolar. This is not correct as they are bipolar. The potential difference is obtained from the exploratory electrode (one of the six chest electrodes) plus the indifferent electrode which is Wilson's central terminal. The precordial leads view the heart in the horizontal and transverse planes. For example lead V6 = the potential measured at the V6 electrode minus a third of the electrodes at the left arm, right arm and left leg:

Lead V6 = V6 − 1/3 (E_R + E_L + E_F)

Clinical tip

In a normal patient when the precordial electrodes and leads are correctly placed and connected, the ECG should show R wave progression increasing in height from V1 to V4. If this pattern is not seen it may be due to pathological changes. However incorrect electrode placement and lead connection should be considered along with the possibility of dextrocardia.

Table 6.2: Orientation of heart viewed by the 12 leads of the standard ECG.

	Region seen	Coronary artery supplying region
I, III, aVF	Inferior surface	Mostly right coronary artery
V1, V2, V3, V4	Anterior surface V1 and V2 are orientated towards the right heart and septum, V3 and V4 face the interventricular septum	Mostly left anterior descending branch of left coronary artery
I, aVL, V5, V6	Left lateral surface I and aVL are orientated towards the high left lateral	Mostly circumflex branch of left coronary artery
aVR	The atria	Branches of main coronary arteries

Table 6.3: Agreed polarity of electrodes in different leads to allow signals to be recorded.

Lead	Positive Pole	Negative Pole
I	Left arm	Right arm
II	Left leg	Right arm
III	Left leg	Left arm
aVR	Right arm	Limb reference
aVL	Left arm	Limb reference
aVF	Left leg (foot)	Limb reference
V1	V1	Chest reference
V2	V2	Chest reference
V3	V3	Chest reference
V4	V4	Chest reference
V5	V5	Chest reference
V6	V6	Chest reference

The established use of 12 defined leads to view the heart was a fundamental aspect of standardising ECG recording. This facilitated research to establish normal values and as a result specific criteria exist to diagnose numerous conditions.

Although the use of 12-leads is now standard practice, this does not mean that it is the ideal configuration. Much more information could be obtained by routinely using additional right sided and posterior leads. This would improve spacial information, sensitivity and specificity for detecting right sided and posterior myocardial infarctions. Attempts have been made to introduce new systems but these have not gained widespread acceptance. New technologies such as cardiac magnetic resonance imaging and computerised tomography have captured the interest of researchers as they can directly visualise structure and function. The ECG can only do this incompletely and indirectly. This does not as yet eliminate the need for standard 12-lead ECGs and as a starting point in the diagnostic process it still remains unsurpassed in terms of speed and cost.

The right leg earth lead

The right leg lead does not take part in the recording of the ECG other than as a safety feature. Theoretically it could be placed anywhere on the body. It is however placed on the right leg just proximal to the ankle and should not be placed anywhere else. If accidental reversal of the leg leads occurs with correct electrode placement there will be little if any change to the ECG recorded. If accidental reversal were to occur if the position of the right leg lead was modified significant changes to the morphology and voltage amplitudes would be recorded.

ECG lead colour codes

When recording an ECG the lead ends are colour coded to aid connection speed. In addition they provide a visual double check to make sure the correct lead is connected to the correct electrode (table 6.4). Correct connection is essential for the ECG equipment to represent the ECG properly in the final tracing. Some ECG machines can recognise when a limb lead has been reversed accidently but the equipment cannot tell if the precordial electrodes are attached to the correct lead. There are two colour code systems in current use. The European system is recommended by the International Electrotechnical Commission (IEC) (2011) and the American system recommended by the Association for the Advancement of Medical Instrumentation (AAMI) and the American Heart Association (AHA, 2007). Ideally all ECG machines across the world should adhere to the same colour code system. This currently does not happen and even within the same country both colour code systems may be in use depending on where the equipment has been manufactured or purchased. In addition to the colour codes, the names of the individual leads also appear on the connection terminal but it should be noted that the written labelling of leads does not always match the colour code. For example, a lead set using the European colour code may have American written labels and vice versa.

Table 6.4:
European and American ECG lead colour codes (N denotes neutral, F foot, V vector, and C chest).

Electrode	Written European code	Colour	Written American code	Colour
Right arm	R	Red	RA	White
Left arm	L	Yellow	LA	Black
Right leg	N	Black	RL	Green
Left leg	F	Green	LL	Red
Fourth intercostal space right sternal border	C1	Red	V1	Red
Fourth intercostal space left sternal border	C2	Yellow	V2	Yellow
Exactly midway between V2 and V4	C3	Green	V3	Green
Fifth intercostal space in the midclavicular line	C4	Brown	V4	Blue
Left anterior axillary line same horizontal plane as V4 (and V6)	C5	Black	V5	Orange
Left midaxillary line same horizontal plane as V4 (and V5)	C6	Purple	V6	Purple

If using an unsealed yoke system, it is possible to purchase additional leads that are not colour coded. Although extremely useful when a broken lead needs to be replaced there is a potential risk of incorrectly attaching the lead to the wrong electrode. This risk is multiplied if more than one non-colour coded lead is used.

The traditional Einthoven and Cabrera or panoramic format

When we look at a typical ECG it is laid out in a standardised pattern with the three Einthoven leads first, the three augmented limb leads second followed thirdly by the six precordial leads. This is a historical arrangement and there is no evidence base to support the practice. It has been proposed that it would be more diagnostically useful to alter this configuration and adopt the Cabrera format also called the panoramic format.

The Cabrera format arranges the order of the limb leads in a more logical manner to make the electrical wavefront progression down the conduction system easier to see. The sequence display order is aVL, I, then -aVR (which is normal aVR but inverted), II, aVF, III, followed by normal six precordial leads from V1 to V6 in numerical order. The main advantage to the Cabrera system is that ischaemia and myocardial infarctions are more easily seen as ST changes even when those changes are subtle (Menown and Adgey, 2000). As with the traditional layout any changes over time may also be compared.

Lead aVR is displayed upside down as this improves diagnosis of inferior and lateral myocardial infarction. Logically it also represents the lead 'missing' between leads II and III moving from left to right or right to left in the hexaxial reference system. Since Cabrera uses the same 10 electrode and electrode positions as the standard ECG, and the only difference is that aVR is inverted by the ECG recording equipment most resistance to its adoption appears to be that the standard format is deeply ingrained in clinical practice however it is beginning to be more widely used in Europe particularly in Sweden. ECG machines are now including the Cabrera and standard layouts in their software.

Summary of key points:

- The ECG patient cable consists of a connection to the electrocardiograph, a yoke, ten patient leads and electrode connectors. Depending on the manufacturer and model individual designs vary.

- Although only ten electrodes are applied to the body, twelve different views of the heart are obtained. The limb leads are required for all twelve views. The six limb leads are derived by combining information from three limb electrodes in different ways. The limb electrodes are again used in Wilson's central terminal to derive the remaining six leads in combination with the six precordial electrodes.

- There are two colour code systems in use, the European and the American. These systems differ and practitioners must be aware of the system used on each electrocardiograph.

- The six limb leads view the heart from the frontal plane, while the six precordial leads view the heart in the horizontal and transverse planes.

- It has been suggested that the ECG should be displayed in the Cabrera format rather than the traditional Einthoven format.

Key review questions

1. When recording an ECG you notice that a poor quality signal is obtained in leads I and III. Using your knowledge of lead derivation explain what is happening.

2. What are the possible consequences of having access to electrocardiographs which use different colour code systems?

3. Convinced by the evidence that the Cabrera format is a more logical layout for displaying ECG information a decision has been made to adopt this system. What organisational implication does this present and how might you address this?

References

Albert, N.M., Hancock, K., Murray, T., Karafa, M., Runner, J.C., Fowler, S.B., Nadeau, C.A., Rice, K.L., Krajewski, S. (2010). 'Cleaned, ready-to-use, reusable electrocardiographic lead wires as a source of pathogenic microorganisms.' *American Journal of Critical Care.* **19**(6): e73–80.

American Heart Association, the American College of Cardiology Foundation; and the Heart Rhythm Society. (2007). 'Recommendations for the standardization and interpretation of the electrocardiogram Part I: The electrocardiogram and its technology.' *Journal of the American College of Cardiology.* **49**(10): 1128–35.

Goldberger, E. (1942a). 'A simple, indifferent, electrocardiographic electrode of zero potential and a technique of obtaining augmented, unipolar, extremity leads.' *American Heart Journal.* **23**(4): 483–92.

Goldberger, E. (1942b). 'The aVR, aVL, and aVF leads. A simplification of standard electrocardiography.' *American Heart Journal.* **24**: 378–96.

International Electrotechnical Commission (IEC) (2011) 'International Standard Medical Electrical Equipment – Part 2-25: Particular requirements for the basic safety and essential performance of electrocardiographs 60601-2-25.' *Annex BB (informative) Electrodes, their positions, identifications and colour codes.* p. 51.

Jancin, B. (2004). 'Antibiotic resistant pathogens found on 77% of ECG lead wires.' *Cardiology News.* **2**(3): 14.

Menown, I.B.A., Adgey, A.A.J. (2000). 'Improving the ECG classification of inferior and lateral myocardial infarction by inversion of lead aVR.' *Heart.* **83**(6): 657–60.

Wilson, F.N., Macleod, A.G., Barker, P.S. (1932). 'Electrocardiographic leads which record potential variations produced by the heart at a single point.' *Proceedings of the Society of Experimental Biology and Medicine.* **29**: 1011–12.

Wilson, F.N., Johnston, F.D., MacLeod, A.G., Barker, P.S. (1934). 'Electrocardiograms that represent the potential variations of a single electrode.' *American Heart Journal.* **9**(4): 447–58.

Chapter 7

Understanding ECG equipment, specification standards and setting choices for recording ECGs

By the end of this chapter you should be able to:
- describe the basic components of the electrocardiograph
- recognise safety issues associated with recording electrocardiographs
- understand the importance of using equipment that meets recommended specification standards
- recognise the importance of quality assurance in ECG recording.

The first commercial electrocardiograph was manufactured by Edelmann and Sons of Munich and was based on Einthoven's adaptation of the string galvanometer. The equipment was cumbersome and required patients to place their lower limbs into a sodium chloride solution contained within glass electrode jars. Although accurate measurements could be made the electrocardiograph's usefulness was limited as it was not portable.

Enhancements to the design began soon after it was first manufactured and a series of improvements resulted in the first portable electrocardiograph being produced toward the end of the 1920s. Modern equipment now makes use of computers and microelectronics but many of the components are similar to those used on these earlier models.

Electrocardiograph components

The modern electrocardiograph is a sophisticated piece of computerised electronic equipment. Typical components include a power supply, input via the patient cable, an analogue to digital converter, amplifiers, filters, graphical display and a recording device. As the electrocardiograph processes very weak signals from the skin surface, any interference will affect the tracing. The equipment must be designed to amplify the weak cardiac signals whilst effectively reducing the unwanted non-cardiac signals.

There are numerous methods to reduce the unwanted signals, however many of these also alter the cardiac signal. As a result standards have been set by the American Heart Association stating recommendations for instrument design and component function. A simplified block diagram is shown in figure 7.1 to illustrate the basic steps required to record an electrocardiogram.

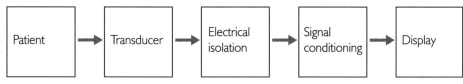

Figure 7.1: Steps required to record an electrocardiogram.

The equipment design must:

- convert the ionic current into an electrical signal
- be electrically safe
- amplify the electrical signal to a clinically useful level
- suppress interference including AC interference (50–60Hz)
- display/record the signals.

Modern machines are more complicated than this. They have data input terminals so that patient demographics can be entered. A keyboard can be used to input patient demographics, an analogue to digital converter is used to digitise the data so that the sophisticated algorithms are incorporated to facilitate the interpretation of the ECG data, and storage capacity is available for large qualities of data. Some are also able to utilise barcode scanners and transmission technology.

Power source

Electrocardiographs are powered by a 50/60Hz AC mains supply. They have the additional capability of being powered by an integral rechargeable battery pack. The battery should be sufficient to deal with a full day's workload if fully charged. Therefore overnight charging is a convenient way of managing battery power.

Clinical tip

Check the user manual in relation to battery management. Some batteries need to be fully discharged and recharged regularly whilst others need to remain fully charged to extend their life.

Safety

It is essential that the electrocardiograph is electrically safe, particularly as the patient may be connected to devices such as drips. An indwelling saline filled catheter would provide a low resistance path to the patient's heart and therefore the potential for a small current to stimulate ventricular fibrillation. It is recommended that any electrocardiograph leakage current is less than ten microamperes (Laks *et al.*, 1996). The electrocardiograph must also be capable of limiting current to this value in the event of fault occurring with the equipment. To address this, an isolation transformer is used as it both protects the patient from equipment faults and the equipment from high energy potentials that may arise for example due to cardiac defibrillation. An isolation transformer provides an interface between the electrical system and the electrocardiograph system and can be used to limit leakage current to the recommended levels.

Transducers

ECG electrodes convert ionic current from the body into electrical current flow. Consequently electrodes act as transducers. It is the electrolyte which has a high ionic concentration that aids in this role. The integrity of the ECG lead attached to the electrode and the input into the electrocardiograph must be maintained for the signals to continue onwards.

Signal conditioning/processing

Once the signals have been acquired they are amplified, filtered and converted from analogue to digital signals. The main sources of artifact in the signals come from electrical, muscle and baseline wander. Artifact is described in detail in chapter 9.

1. Instrumentation Amplifier

An instrumentation amplifier is used to boost the weak cardiac signal detected by the electrodes. It is important when increasing the size of the ECG signal not to also increase any unwanted signals (artifact) at the same time. Enhancement of the weak ECG signal while reducing artifact is accomplished by using high input impedance and common mode rejection ratio. Common mode voltage or artifact is any AC or DC signals that are common to both of the electrodes and therefore both the positive and negative ends of the instrumentation amplifier. It is important to remove this artifact as it results in spurious data being obtained. After amplification by the instrumentation amplifier a high pass filter is used. An additional method of removing common mode artifact is to use a driven right leg circuit (page 93).

2. High and low frequency cut off filters

The AHA (2007) recommended a setting of 0.05Hz for the low frequency cut off and 150Hz for the high frequency cut-off when recording adult electrocardiograms. For children the high cut off will need to be increased depending on heart rate. 250Hz is frequently used in the paediatric setting. Using these settings will minimise any distortion to the ECG signal and maintain its diagnostic quality.

3. Analogue to digital conversion

The ECG data obtained from the body surface is in analogue form. However in order to analyse the signals using computer based systems, to digitally store the ECG, or transmit the ECG to another location the analogue signals must be converted to digital signals. Analogue to digital converters sample the ECG voltage signals at timed intervals. These intervals must be close enough together to prevent any information being missed. This is known as the sampling frequency. The different ECG voltages are assigned a number or code for each voltage measured usually using one of five possible methods:

- Counter
- Tracking
- Dual slope
- Successive approximation
- Flash

Whatever method is used signal fidelity must be maintained. Fidelity is the measure of distortion to the ECG waves and intervals when they are processed and converted from analogue to digital signals. High fidelity ECG machines produce less distortion. The AHA (2007) recommended oversampling of the analogue signal to provide the recommended bandwidth in the digitised signal.

Fidelity is also important in the storage of digital ECGs which require compression to save storage space. When decompressed for viewing again they must remain undistorted. The degree of fidelity required depends upon what will happen to the data produced. If ECGs are being manually read then a very small variation difference in the voltages pre and post processing is acceptable. If ECGs are being analysed by computer based systems greater fidelity is required.

Notch filters

A notch filter removes a particular frequency from an ECG signal. These filters are practitioner deployed and found on the electrocardiograph control panel. The use of the notch filters is not recommended and they should only be used after all other action to reduce artifact has been unsuccessful (SCST, 2010). The use of notch filters should not be considered a routine part of recording a standard 12-lead ECG, as they distort the waveforms recorded. It is recommended that the electrocardiograph should automatically alert the user if a notch filter is used and that the filter is automatically disengaged between recordings (Kligfield & Okin, 2007).

Filtered ECGs are sometimes incorrectly assumed to be good quality due to the absence of artifact. However, the use of the 40 Hz muscle artifact filter can affect the similar frequency signals found in an ECG. This results in ECG waveform distortion (SCST, 2010). The ECG shown in figure 7.2 below illustrates the effects of using a 40Hz filter to remove muscle artifact. Whilst the changes caused by the filter are subtle in this normal example, there is still a loss of R and S wave height and flattening of the T wave in lead I and a flattened ST segment and slurring of the T wave in lead II. Similar changes occurred throughout the whole ECG. In this case this would not have been enough to change the clinical interpretation overall, however in some patients flattening of the ST segment and T waves may be enough to misdiagnose ischaemia.

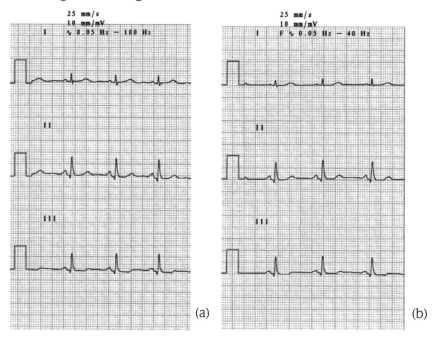

(a)   (b)

Figure 7.2: (a) ECG recorded without filter selected (b) same ECG recorded using a 40 Hz muscle artifact filter.

Signal analysis

The electrocardiograph contains a microprocessor for signal analysis. Complex algorithm software is used to analyse the data, make measurements and produce a computer generated report. The AHA (2007) recommended standardisation of global measurement algorithms and Mason *et al.* (2007) in an effort to promote a homogeneous diagnostic code set produced a list of ECG diagnostic terms. Adoption of these diagnostic terms globally will ensure consistency in ECG interpretation.

Display device/recording device

The final ECG signals may be displayed on a high resolution liquid crystal display (LCD) screen. This feature increases the economical use of the equipment as a good quality signal can be identified on each of the leads before recording and printing. Measurements should not be made from the screen as it is not accurately calibrated. ECGs are printed in hardcopy form on specialised medical graph paper. This is ruled with one millimetre divisions along the time and voltage axes, with every fifth division ruled darker. The dimensional accuracies of this recording paper must not deviate by more than 1 per cent when used in temperatures between 10 and 50 degrees centigrade. Printer types include thermal dot array and ink jet formats.

Input of additional data

Patient demographics are entered via a keyboard system. To optimise input speed standard alphanumeric keyboards are used. Some of the latest designs incorporate a bar code scanner to further improve clinical efficiency. Although the ECG can be recorded without patient demographic information being entered this is not advisable as failure to manually enter the data once the recording has been completed will render the ECG as useless.

Equipment specifications

Because the ECG can be affected by how the voltages are measured, processed and represented in graphical form, equipment for clinical use needs to meet a set of performance specifications. The current specifications were updated in 2007 (ANSI/AAMI, 2007). The specifications relate to the manufacturing of the equipment and equipment use. The specifications set minimum standards for accurate acquisition of electrocardiographic data. It is essential that the practitioner is actively involved in the departmental quality assurance programme. Routine monitoring, evaluation and servicing of the electrocardiograph will help to ensure accurate data is recorded.

The practitioner should ensure that the integrity of the equipment and measurable specifications such as calibration are checked at regular intervals. Some parameters can only be checked when the equipment is serviced.

Equipment setting checks

Switch on self-test

Most systems complete a self-test when switched on. Routines followed during this self-test are determined by the manufacture, but commonly include checks for battery voltage, memory capacity, software errors and the printer status. An error code is normally displayed if any of the routines identifies a fault. Depending on the code this can either be addressed by the practitioner or will require contact with a service engineer.

Sensitivity, gain, calibration or standardisation

Sensitivity or gain refers to the recorded response of the ECG machine to an applied voltage. All ECG machines are adjusted at manufacture so that a 1 millivolt signal applied for 0.2 seconds will produce a 10mm deflection on the ECG recorded lasting for five small squares. Setting the equipment sensitivity or gain so that it records the expected deflection on the input of a known impulse is called calibration or standardisation (figure 7.3). Sensitivity should also be checked at 5mm/mV, 20mm/mV and any other setting the ECG machine is capable of. The sensitivity is adjusted to meet this criterion. All ECG machines are required to send a calibration signal producing a square waveform in the ECG at some point throughout the tracing. Typically this happens at the start or end of the ECG and is called a calibration signal. It should be checked in every ECG recorded to make sure it measures 10mm high and 5mm wide when the standard recording settings are being used.

Sensitivity, calibration, standardisation or gain drift

An ECG machine must be able to hold its calibration settings over long periods of time otherwise they do not hold their accuracy and are unsuitable for clinical use.

Modern ECG machines have very high levels of sensitivity stability maintaining their calibration setting within permitted variation levels for up to one year or more. In order to meet specifications sensitivity drift is measured in one minute and over a one hour period. A known voltage is applied to the input of the ECG machine and then measured at the output over the extended period of time. In one minute the voltage should not drift by more than $\pm 0.33\%$ per minute. Over one hour the overall net change should not be greater than $\pm 3\%$. The test for sensitivity drift is repeated for each calibration setting the ECG machine is capable of, e.g., 5mm/mV, 10mm/mV and 20mm/mV.

For an ECG to be diagnostic each of the 12 leads and their constituent waveforms must not overlap and be clear enough to measure voltage directly from the graph. If waveforms are not clearly separated it is necessary to temporarily change the relationship of the voltage input to voltage output, or the paper speed to see what is happening in the ECG. For example, if the QRS complexes are high voltage and overlapping, the voltage setting at which the ECG is recorded should be reduced to half voltage (5mm = 1mV), so that each QRS may be clearly seen and measured. It is poor practice to modify voltage across the whole ECG unless required. Voltage is most frequently altered in the precordial leads and the electrocardiograph typically permits altering the voltage setting in these leads whilst maintaining the standard setting in the limb leads. However if voltage needs to be altered in the limb leads most equipment settings require the complete ECG to be recorded at this setting. Any deviation from the standard calibration should be clearly annotated on the ECG.

It is recommended that two ECGs are produced, one using the standard voltage, and the other at the changed voltage settings. Both ECGs should be annotated clearly and kept together in the patient chart. It is important to make sure that any changes in the ECG machine settings are returned to normal at the end of the recording prior to use on the next patient.

When the voltage calibration settings are changed on modern ECG machines each voltage will produce its own characteristic square wave or box shaped calibration signal. Some examples are shown in figure 7.3 The practitioner must be able to look at the calibration box signal to verify changes made in the calibration setting, or if interpreting an ECG, be able to recognise what settings were used to prevent misinterpretation.

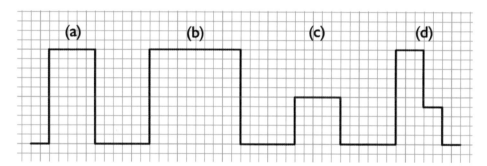

Figure 7.3: The standard 12-lead ECG calibration signal appears as a 10mm high by 5mm wide box when calibration is correctly set at:
(a) 1mV = 10mm and paper speed at 25mm/second
(b) Paper speed at 50mm/second
(c) Limb and chest leads at half voltage (5mm = 1mV)
(d) Limb leads at standard voltage (10mm = 1mV), chest leads at half voltage (5mm = 1mV)

Over and under damping

The standard calibration signal should be 10mm high and 5mm wide with a sharp right angled waveform. When the ECG machine is not properly adjusted the standardisation can be over or under damped. Over damping occurs when the stylus is lying too tightly against the ECG paper producing high friction inertia. Quick accurate movement of the stylus is reduced due to friction against the paper and the ECG calibration signal appears curved at the corners. It may also occur when the ink jet is not responsive enough to sudden changes in voltage. An over damped ECG machine may record artifactual ST segment changes. Under damping occurs when the stylus is set too loosely against the paper. This produces a spike on top of the beginning of the calibration signal. It is caused as the stylus shoots past where it should stop as friction against the paper is reduced. It can also occur when the inkjet sprays past its expected limits. Under damping makes fast moving ECG waves such as the QRS appear larger than they actually are.

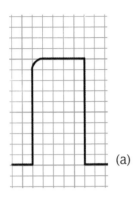 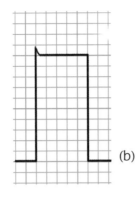

(a) (b) *Figure 7.4: (a) Over damping and (b) under damping visible in the calibration signal.*

Input dynamic range

This specification tests the ability of the ECG machine to react and accurately record fast changes in electrical potentials. Fast voltage changes occur in the ECG during the QRS complex and particularly when the patient is in tachycardia. The specification requires that an ECG machine can measure fast voltage changes clearly on paper and on a screen if available between –5mV and +5mV occurring at a rate of 320mV/sec at a gain setting of 5mm/mV. When the gain is increased above 5mm/mV the tracing obtained should still be clearly visible.

Time intervals and time base accuracy

ECGs must run at a known speed for timing measurements to be accurate. ECG machines are required to be able to print time constant markers on ECG paper. These are marks produced at one second intervals or less, so that paper speed can be checked. An accuracy of ±2% is permitted. In some clinical settings paper speed is rarely checked but as it is a vital part of the calibration process this should be verified routinely. Another way to verify paper speed is to start recording in manual mode. Then using a stop watch mark the paper at ten second intervals. The number of squares between the marks are counted and multiplied by six so that the paper speed can be calculated since paper speed can be changed to look for example at waveforms more clearly. This particularly applies to P waves that might not be visible until paper speed is increased spreading the waves out. Or paper speed may be changed to record over an extended period of time without producing volumes of paper. Time intervals should therefore be checked at 25mm/sec, 12.5mm/ sec and 50mm/sec etc. Any change from standard should be clearly annotated on the ECG and the original plus the altered ECG filed in the patient notes.

Frequency response

Frequency response defines the ability of the ECG equipment to accurately record both fast and slow moving waveforms. QRS complexes are considered to be high frequency waves or fast waves and T waves are low frequency or slow waves. The frequency response of a system can be measured by applying a 1mV alternating sinusoidal input of differing frequencies and measuring the response. This procedure is normally carried out by the service engineer.

Linearity

Linearity refers to the ability to produce a deflection maintaining the calibration ratio over a wide variety of input voltages. In other words if a signal of direct current 1mV is input a deflection of 10mm is produced, 2mV will cause a deflection of 20mm and 3mV a deflection of 30mm and so on. The response recorded should always be directly proportional to the applied voltage. The variation over the entire recording range of the ECG machine should not vary by more than ±5%.

Safety Tests

This will include earth leakage testing which is usually measured with normal and reversed mains polarity, protective earth resistance and leads leakage current. The maximum leakage current limits are defined in the 2011 edition of International Electrotechnical Commission 60601-1. However the American Heart Association Committee on Electrocardiography recommend that current leakage should be limited to 10 microamperes in no fault or single fault conditions (Laks *et al.*, 1996).

Summary of key points:

- The electrocardiograph requires a power source. Components within the electrocardiograph amplify the small cardiac voltages whilst reducing common mode artifact. By using an analogue to digital converter the data can be analysed and a report produced.

- The electrocardiograph must be designed to ensure patient safety. It is powered by an isolated main supply, in addition the interface between the patient and the electrocardiograph components is also isolated. This provides protection for the patient, practitioner and the internal components.

- Adhering to established standards improves the accuracy and clinical usefulness of the electrocardiogram.

- A quality assurance programme is necessary to ensure electrocardiograph equipment is meeting recommended standards.

Key review questions

1. What does a common-mode rejection ratio measure?

2. Why does the American Heart Association Committee on Electrocardiography recommend that current leakage should be limited to 10 microamperes in no fault or single fault conditions

3. What would happen to the ECG if the recommended filter settings were not used?

References

American Heart Association, American College of Cardiology foundation; and the Heart Rhythm Society (2007). 'Recommendations for the standardization and interpretation of the electrocardiogram Part I: The electrocardiogram and its technology.' *Journal of the American College of Cardiology* **49**(10): 1128–35.

American National Standards Institute (2007). Diagnostic electrocardiographic devices (ANSI/AAMI EC11:1991/(R)2001/(R)2007). Arlington, VA: Association for the Advancement of Medical Instrumentation.

Kligfield P., Okin, P.M. (2007). 'Prevalence and clinical implications of improper filter settings in routine electrocardiography'. *American Journal of Cardiology.* **99**(5): 711–13.

Laks, M., Arzbaecher, R., Bailey, J.J., Geselowitz, D.B., Berson, A.S. (1996). 'Recommendations for safe current limits for electrocardiographs: a statement for healthcare professionals from the committee on electrocardiography, American Heart Association'. *Circulation.* **93**: 837–9.

Mason, J.W., Hancock, E.W., Gettes, L. (2007). 'Recommendations for the standardization and interpretation of the electrocardiogram, part II: electrocardiography diagnostic statement list: a scientific statement from the American Heart Association Electrocardiography and Arrhythmias Committee, Council on Clinical Cardiology; the American College of Cardiology Foundation; and the Heart Rhythm Society.' *Circulation.* **115**: 1325–32.

Society of Cardiological Science and Technology (2010) Clinical Guidelines by Consensus: Recording a Standard 12-lead ECG: An Approved Methodology. Available from:
http://www.scst.org.uk/resources/consensus_guideline_for_recording_a_12_lead_ecg_Rev_072010b.pdf (Accessed 6/3/12).

Chapter 8

Recording and checking the ECG

By the end of this chapter you should be able to:
- prepare the equipment and patient prior to recording the ECG
- understand the importance of providing support for the patient to obtain a diagnostic quality ECG
- appreciate a range of situations where standard electrode positioning cannot be achieved and understand how to correctly modify electrode placements
- understand the benefits of having an ECG recording protocol.

The ECG is an essential tool in the diagnosis and management of a wide range of conditions. Its accuracy in recording true clinical changes depends upon the use of equipment that meets clinical specifications (see chapter 7). Good preparation of the equipment and patient along with obtaining a tracing from standardised electrode positions are all equally important in recording a diagnostic quality ECG.

Recording an ECG

1. Equipment preparation for recording an ECG
Being organised will save both time and contribute to the effective running of the electrocardiographic service. Before using an electrocardiograph check that it is clean and all the cables and outer casings are intact and show no signs of damage. Plug the electrocardiograph into the power supply or check the battery has been charged. Switch on the machine and allow it to complete a self-test. Once the equipment passes the self-test, it is ready for use. If a problem is identified during set up, this should be rectified. If the fault does not allow this, the equipment should be labelled with a description of the problem. The equipment should also be removed from use and the departmental protocol for informing the service engineer followed.

Sufficient disposable supplies should be available for recording the ECG including:
- Electrodes
- Gauze
- Mild soap solution
- Preparation pads
- Alcohol impregnated wipes
- Hand decontamination products
- Gloves
- ECG paper
- Clippers
- Gowns
- Tissues
- Paper roll

2. Preparation of the patient for recording an ECG
When a patient is referred to an ECG service there should always be a fully completed request form. An example is provided in figure 8.1. Age, gender, race and medications can cause variations in the ECG recorded. These details must be complete on the ECG request form so that they may be taken into consideration when reporting.

Electrocardiography (ECG) request form

Organisation logo

Patient Details:

Title: (Mr/Mrs/Miss/Ms)   Medications: _____

Surname: _____   _____

Forename: _____   _____

Address: _____   _____

_____   Male/Female BP _____

Postcode: _____   Height: _____

DOB: _____   Weight: _____

ID#: _____   Race: _____

Reason for referral:	**Risk Factors**	Y	N
	Diabetes	☐	☐
	Hypertension	☐	☐
	Smoker/Ex-smoker	☐	☐
	Positive Family History	☐	☐
	Raised Cholesterol	☐	☐

Referrer's name:

Contact details

If patient is given their request form to bring to the department provide details of location and contact number here

---

Figure 8.1: Example ECG form.

Good patient communication reduces patient anxiety and therefore should help to improve patient cooperation and the quality of the ECG recorded. An ECG patient information leaflet is an ideal way of enhancing communication before the patient attends as it provides information about the test, why it is performed and how the patient may obtain their results. Patient information leaflets are intended to be an initial source of information preparing the patient for their appointment and allowing them to think of any questions they may like addressed when they attend. They are not intended to be the sole source of information and do not replace information given by a practitioner face-to-face. Patient details are checked on arrival to confirm identity. The following pages show an example of an ECG patient information leaflet.

[Logo]

[Practice name]

[Practice address and main contact number]

Electrocardiography (ECG) Patient Information Leaflet

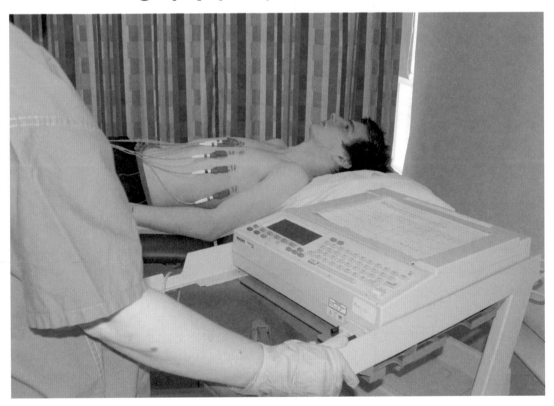

Version 1, April 2012

Review date: May 2016

You have been referred for an ECG. This leaflet will provide you with information about the procedure and help you prepare for your appointment

What is an ECG?

An ECG is a quick, painless procedure which helps the doctor to make a diagnosis. Each time the heart muscle contracts and relaxes it produces tiny electrical signals which can be measured using electrodes placed on the surface of the body. The ECG machine picks up the electrical signals and turns them into a printed graph.

Why is an ECG necessary?

There are many reasons for recording an ECG such as chest pain or palpitations. ECGs may also be performed if another condition is present such as diabetes, before an operation or to rule out a disease.

What happens during the test?

You will be asked to remove all clothing from the upper body and to expose the lower legs and arms. You will be given a gown to wear and asked to lie on an examination couch. The skin will be cleaned and sticky electrodes placed on carefully located positions. It is sometimes necessary to shave small areas to remove hair. You will be asked to relax and lie still whilst the recording is made.

Will the test tell the doctor what is wrong?

An ECG is a very useful clinical tool, however further tests may be required to obtain sufficient information to make a diagnosis.

Are there any side effects?

The ECG is a painless and harmless investigation. On very rare occasions the electrodes may cause a temporary reddening of the skin or an allergic reaction at the electrode sites. If you have any known allergies you should discuss this with the practitioner.

Do I need to make any preparations?

You do not need to make any special preparations for your ECG. If you are on any medication please bring a list with you as some medications can affect the interpretation of the ECG.

When will I know the results?

Test results will be sent to your general practitioner. You should contact your general practitioner approximately seven days after the appointment.

Giving your consent for the procedure

Before the test begins the practitioner will explain the ECG investigation in detail. It is your right to make a decision based on the information given as to whether you wish to proceed or not. You should feel free to ask any questions you might have. Consent is given for an ECG verbally. When you consent you will also be asked to give permission for data sharing. To send your report to your general practitioner, to seek a second opinion or to request past clinical data we need permission to share identifiable patient data with other relevant organisations. We are also required to supply ECG samples for clinical audit and quality assurance.

The hospital operates a strict policy regarding confidentiality, which means your information is never shared with anyone that does not need to know about your clinical condition.

As this is a teaching hospital students will sometimes be present. You will be asked if you are happy for students to watch and/or take part in the test. It is your right to refuse.

Additional assistance

Please notify us if you require additional assistance for your appointment. This may include the need for an interpreter, a wheelchair or any special requirements due to your condition. If you are unsure if additional assistance is needed please feel free to contact us on [insert].

The feedback and complaints procedure

The hospital welcomes both good and bad feedback about your experience. We recognise that monitoring comments helps us to continuously improve. Feedback forms are available from the ECG waiting area. If you have a complaint about any aspect of the service you have received you can:

- Discuss it with the department manager [insert name] during your visit.
- Call the patient care team telephone [insert].
- Write to the quality manager, name, address, telephone number [insert].
- Use the [name of practice] complaints procedure on our website [insert link].

Contacting us:

If you need to change your appointment please contact the appointments office on telephone number [insert]

If you would like to ask a question about the procedure or have any other queries please contact the ECG department telephone [insert]

Text phone/Minicom contact [insert]

Please arrive 15 minutes before your appointment time; if you are late we may need to reschedule your test. Please allow 30 minutes for completion of your appointment.

The hospital operates a strict no smoking policy in all public areas.

The ECG procedure is explained in detail and any questions addressed, once consent has been obtained the patient will need to undress prior to the ECG being recorded. The patient's dignity must be maintained at all time. This will include keeping doors or curtains closed and giving the patient privacy to undress. A front opening gown or sheet should be available so that the patient can cover their chest area once clothing has been removed. This will help the patient relax and reduce the incidence of muscle artifact in the recording.

At the clinic

What information do you currently give to patients regarding ECGs?

Is the same information given to inpatients and outpatients?

In which format is the information presented?

Does this meet the needs of all your patients and is the information equitable?

The checked patient details such as name, age, sex, referring physician etc. are typed into the electrocardiograph in preparation for recording. By entering the details now, if there is something urgent in the ECG the possibility of having an unidentified ECG is prevented. Following patient positioning the practitioner should wash their hands and put on gloves (see table 8.1). The patient's skin is prepared carefully (chapter 4) and the electrodes applied to the limbs and chest in the correct anatomical positions (chapter 3). For inpatients, if the individual is connected to an ECG monitor the monitor electrodes may have to be moved to access the correct 12-lead electrode positions. ECG electrodes should not be placed to avoid monitoring electrodes.

3. Obtaining an ECG recording
The ECG leads are connected to the corresponding electrodes and the patient cable laid gently on top or to the side of the patient. Leads should be slack and not pulling. Check the patient is warm and comfortable, ask them to relax and remain still during the recording. The correct calibration and filter setting is selected and the ECG recorded either manually or using the automatic mode. When the electrocardiograph has a LCD screen the quality of all signals should be confirmed before the ECG is recorded.

4. Post recording
Confirmation of correct calibration is obtained by examining the signal on the tracing. Patient demographics are also rechecked. The 12 leads are examined for quality and lack of artifact. If there is a fault in the ECG or the quality is poor, the ECG is repeated. The ECG is checked for important abnormalities that would require immediate attention. Once diagnostic suitability has been established and no further recordings are required, the leads are disconnected and the electrodes removed. Any remaining electrolyte is wiped off the patient's skin before dressing. If the patient was experiencing symptoms at the time of recording this should be annotated on the ECG. Information regarding the process of obtaining the results is explained. The ECG is dispatched as appropriate.

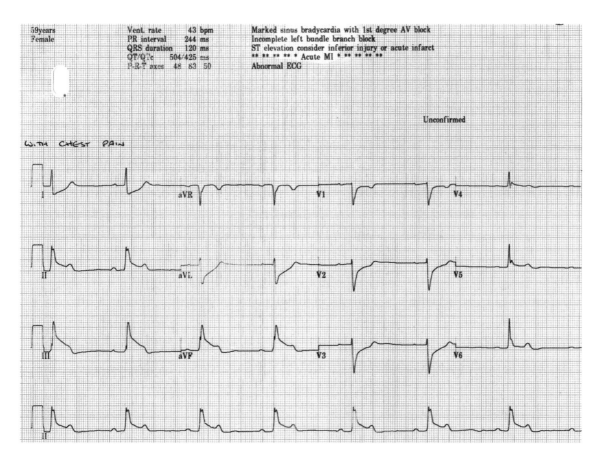

Figure 8.2: Appropriately annotated ECG recorded during symptoms of chest pain.

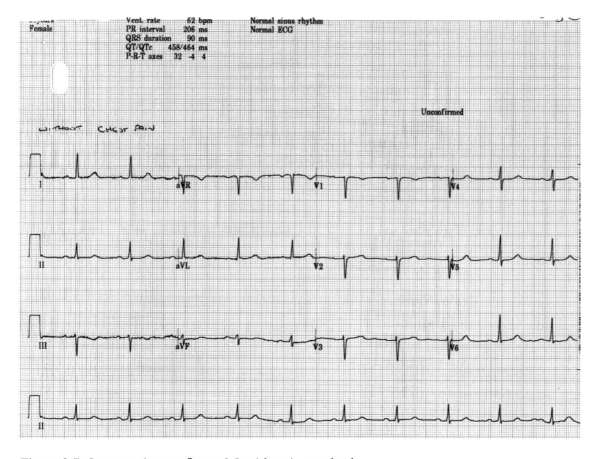

Figure 8.3: Same patient as figure 8.2 with pain resolved.

The ECGs in figures 8.2 and 8.3 were recorded 30 minutes apart. The fact that the first ECG was annotated clearly with the patient's symptoms helps to account for the significant changes between the two tracings. Without clear identification and symptom annotation it is possible that the first tracing may be treated as not belonging to the patient. In this case the blood troponin level was normal and the patient was diagnosed with Prinzmetal angina.

Clinical tip

Annotate the ECG clearly with any alterations made and the reason required, even if the alterations seem insignificant, as it can result in confusion and mismanagement at a future date.

What constitutes a diagnostic quality ECG?

A diagnostic quality ECG is one that has been recorded:

- by an electrocardiograph that meets AHA specifications
- on an electrocardiograph that has been correctly maintained
- using quality ECG graph paper
- by a competent practitioner who has used the standard anatomical positions
- at correct calibration settings
- without external filters (and correct internal filters)
- with clearly identifiable waveforms that do not overlap
- without artifact
- and correctly labelled.

Any tracing that does not meet all the above criteria, although it may in some cases look appropriate, will not be accurate and therefore cannot be used for diagnostic purposes.

The ECG protocol

As the demand for ECGs increase, the range of settings in which they are recorded has become more diverse. Although best practice guidelines for ECG recording exist, their interpretation and implementation vary depending on staff training and experience.

Practitioners who undertake ECG recordings must ensure that they practice within their professional body guidelines, codes of conduct and within the limits of their professional capability. Practitioners must be competent in all aspects of ECG recording. This is achieved through initial training and maintaining continual professional development (CPD) in the area (see chapter 14).

A protocol or standard operating procedure is an additional means of ensuring consistency and quality in ECG recording. Protocols are detailed written instructions that define the steps required to maintain standardisation and complete a procedure such as an ECG. They document the way activities are to be performed to record an ECG. As protocols are written they circumvent the opportunity for miscommunication of information and help to provide a mechanism for audit.

Table 8.1 Typical ECG recording protocol

Action	Rationale
1. Prepare the room where appropriate for recording an ECG	All equipment and disposables should be ready for use as this facilitates smooth running of the service and projects a professional image
2. Prepare the ECG equipment	All clinical equipment must be in clean and safe working order before use
3. Introduction and check patient ID	Patients need to know who is involved in their care and may not always be able to read a name badge. The practitioner needs to confirm the procedure and patient
4. Explain the procedure	For valid consent the patient must have a full understanding of the procedure
5. Answer questions and check if they wish to have a chaperone present during recording	Ensures the patient understands the procedure. The patient may be more relaxed if a chaperone is present
6. Obtain informed consent	Respects the patient's autonomy.
7. Enter patient details into the ECG machine	Identifies the ECG's source and allows the computerised report to be more accurate
8. Give patient privacy to undress	Maintains patient dignity
9. Maintain dignity and keep the patient covered	It is essential to maintain dignity throughout the whole procedure
10. Decontaminate hands and glove-up	Maintains infection control and prevents health acquired infection
11. Ensure the patient is comfortable in a supine position	Ensures patient comfort in the standard position and optimal recording quality
12. Locate and prepare skin at electrode sites	Removes the stratum corneum under the electrode ensuring good contact, minimising artifact and reducing skin impedance.
13. Relocate electrode sites and apply electrodes	Identifies correct electrode positions and facilitates recording
14. Securely attach leads to corresponding electrodes	Facilitates the ECG recording
15. Confirm electrode positions and lead connections	Ensures accuracy
16. Ensure leads are not pulling or tangled	Minimises artifact and prevents leads/electrodes being dislodged
17. Ensure the patient is warm and ask them to relax	Ensures patient comfort and minimises muscle artifact
18. Ask the patient not to talk or move during the recording	To obtain an optimal recording the patient must remain still

19. Record the ECG	To obtain the ECG recording
20. Check the ECG for correct calibration, patient details, date and time	Ensures the recording is standardised and correct details are provided so that it can be used for reference
21. Check the ECG is free of artifact	Ensures diagnostic quality
22. If artifact is present identify source, and re-record	Obtains an optimal diagnostic recording
23. Once a satisfactory tracing has been obtained disconnect leads	Maintains dignity and shows respect for the patient
24. Remove electrodes, clean off any remaining electrolyte and dispose of any used materials	Limits possible reaction to electrolyte and maintains infection control.
25. Give the patient privacy to dress	Maintains dignity
26. Remove gloves and decontaminate hands	Maintains infection control and prevents healthcare acquired infection
27. Inform the patient how the report is obtained and address any questions	Reassures the patient and keeps them informed.
28. Ensure ECG reaches relevant destination	Ensures the ECG information is acted upon
29. Archive copy as per department protocol	Ensures a copy is available for future reference
30. Complete departmental investigation log	Facilitates patient contact if a problem is identified with the equipment
31. Glove up, clean equipment and follow departmental decontamination procedures if necessary	Maintains infection control
32. Remove gloves and decontaminate hands	Maintains infection control

At the clinic

ECGs and the patient voice

Patient-centred care puts the voice of the patient at the heart of healthcare provision. Listening and being responsive to individual's needs ensures that the patient's voice guides the ECG recording process. The comments below have been made by patients who have experienced ECG recording:

The doctor told me my heart rate was fast but it can be daunting having an ECG and no one seemed to notice I was stressed.'

'I didn't realise I had to undress for an ECG, that was embarrassing enough but I was wearing an old bra and that made me feel even worse.'

'I spent a fortune on my fake tan, and the nurse rubbed it off and didn't even say why.'

'They kept telling me to relax but I could hear the patient talking in the next bed and staff kept entering my cubicle and not properly closing the curtains. How do they expect you to relax with all that going on?'

Many of the above patient comments may be familiar to you. If these comments were made in relation to your practice how might you address the issues raised?

How do you currently collect feedback from patients and can this be improved?

What are the benefits and limitations of engaging with the patient voice?
To what extent do you feel your workplace supports the patient voice?

Summary of key points

- ECG equipment should be prepared before starting to record an ECG. This establishes the equipment is safe to use and the proper settings have been selected.

- Whilst preparing the patient it is imperative that they are respected and their dignity is maintained at all times. Explaining the procedure in a calm and confident manner will not only provide the patient with the necessary information but will also help reassure them. If the patient is relaxed a good quality tracing should be obtained.

- When designing an ECG request form for your service it is important to consider the information required to ensure an accurate diagnosis and identification of the patient.

- A range of clinical situations may be encountered where standard electrode positioning cannot be achieved and it is necessary to modify electrode placements. Any deviation from the standard recording must be annotated on the ECG.

- A protocol for recording ECGs is good practice because it ensures consistency and quality.

Key review questions

1. What are the key points that should be included when describing the ECG process to a patient?

2. Why as a practitioner recording an ECG should you project a calm confident manner?

3. Why is an unlabelled ECG non-diagnostic?

Chapter 9

Recognising and reducing artifact in the ECG recording

By the end of this chapter you should be able to:

- demonstrate an understanding of the consequences associated with using a poor quality artifactual ECG
- recognise a wide range of ECG artifacts
- identify the steps required to reduce or eliminate these artifacts in an ECG recording
- apply theoretical knowledge to improve the quality of ECGs recorded in the clinical environment.

ECG Artifact

All cells in the body are excitable. In other words they are capable of producing electrical potentials. This occurs as a result of electrochemical changes between the inside and outside of the cell as electrically charged ions such as sodium (Na^+), potassium (K^+) and chloride (Cl^-) move across the cell membrane. The cells exhibit a resting electrical potential and when appropriately stimulated they produce an action potential. It is the summation of the electrical changes that we measure in the ECG at the body surface. It is created as the cells of the cardiac conduction system and myocardium are stimulated and depolarise (create an action potential) then repolarise (return to their resting state). The electrical signals are very small, normally 0.0001 to 0.003 Volts (V) and have a frequency of 0.05 to 100 Hertz (Hz) or cycles per second (Smith, 1984; Bailey *et al.*, 1990).

When recording an ECG it is the cardiac activity that is of interest and not electrical signals from other parts of the body, equipment or the environment. Any unwanted electrical signals which interfere with and distort the true cardiac signals are called artifact. Artifact is a common problem in electrocardiography and there are many different types but all reduce the diagnostic quality of the ECG. Once artifact has been identified appropriate action should be taken to rectify or reduce the level so that an interpretation of the ECG data may be made with confidence. This protects the patient from misdiagnosis and mismanagement. It has been established that ECG artifact results in interpreting false pathological changes as arrhythmias and ischaemic disease (Chase and Brady, 2000). It can also lead to miscalculating the heart rate and cardiac axis. The ability to recognise and rectify artifactual problems is fundamental to achieving competency in recording ECGs, a fact supported by the major ECG guidelines (SCST, 2010, ACC/AHA 2001). One reason why recognition and elimination of artifact is so important is clearly illustrated by a survey conducted by Knight *et al.* in 2001. When 766 doctors were shown an ECG with artifact mimicking wide QRS complex tachycardia only 6 per cent of internists, 42 per cent of cardiologists and 62 per cent of cardiac electrophysiologists correctly identified the tracing as artifact even though partial sinus QRSs could be seen dispersed through the tracing. This should have alerted the participants to the presence of artifact. When accurate urgent diagnoses are required the ability to separate artifact from true cardiac arrhythmias is vital. In non-emergency situations the ability to detect artifact is just as great. The normal management for ventricular tachycardia episodes which are non-sustained is electrophysiological testing. Thus an initial misdiagnosis may lead to unnecessary and potentially dangerous investigations. An earlier study by Knight *et al.* in 1999 published in the *New England Journal of Medicine* had previously highlighted this fact. Not only does artifact mimic fatal arrhythmias, it can also distort the ECG to appear as other arrhythmias and make the analysis of the waveforms difficult or impossible.

Fortunately ECG artifacts have very characteristic patterns which with care and attention are easily recognised. Artifact may arise in one or two leads, or in multiple leads. Multiple lead artifact is more dangerous as it can mimic arrhythmias such as atrial fibrillation or flutter, ventricular fibrillation and ventricular tachycardia as the true waves are obscured throughout the whole ECG (Salerno *et al.*, 2003; Vereckei, 2004). Artifact arises from two main sources, physiological and non-physiological.

Physiological sources of artifact

1. Electromyogenic artifact also known as muscle or somatic tremor

The electrical signals produced by cardiac muscle are relatively small. Signals produced by skeletal muscle are called electromyogenic or EMG signals. EMG signals are much larger in amplitude and frequency than the cardiac potentials. They appear as spikes at irregular intervals and heights. When cardiac and skeletal muscle signals are picked up by the electrocardiograph the P, Q, R, S and T waves cannot be clearly seen in the resulting tracing. EMG artifact may be intermittent as the patient briefly moves or continuous as the patient is unable to relax a group of muscles. EMG artifact is known to cause changes in the ECG which can mimic fatal arrhythmias such as ventricular tachycardia (Srikureja *et al.*, 2000). The artifact caused by Parkinson's disease is frequently mistaken for atrial flutter or fibrillation as it is relatively low in amplitude and occurs at a characteristic frequency of 3–5 Hertz (Hz) (Hwang, 2008). Occasionally it can mimic a more serious arrhythmia. In 2005 Bhatia and Turner identified a series of patients with Parkinson's disease whose ECGs contained EMG artifact which was subsequently misdiagnosed and treated as ventricular tachycardia. The unnecessary treatment ranged from a simple precordial thump to the more serious intervention of an implantable cardioverter defibrillator.

Electromyogenic artifact stops or reduces when the skeletal muscles relax. Therefore patient relaxation should be the primary focus in any attempt to remove or reduce this artifact in the ECG. However there are special circumstances in which this might not be possible including where the patient has a tremor due to underlying disease. Since the EMG spikes are so very different from the ECG waveforms they may be reduced by filtering, but this distorts the ECG and should only be used as a last resort at the recommended filtering levels (SCST, 2010; ACC/AHA 2001). The presence of tremor during an ECG recording and any use of filters should always be clearly annotated on the graph (figure 9.1).

A special type of EMG artifact called respiratory artifact (not to be confused with respiratory swing artifact discussed later in this chapter) is in fact clinically useful as it provides important physiological data. It is associated with high risk increased work of breathing caused by compromised cardiac or pulmonary function (Littman *et al.*, 2008). It is seen in the ECG as short bursts of EMG artifact which occur every time the patient inspires.

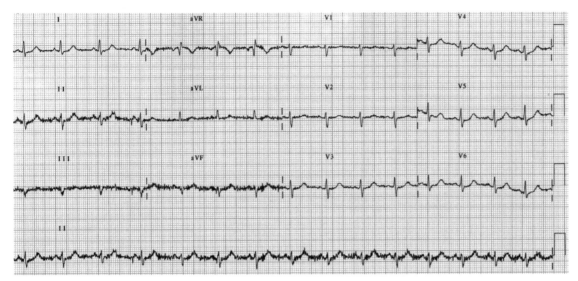

Figure 9.1: Electromyogenic artifact.

Table 9.1: Steps to limit or remove myogenic artifact.

Electromyogenic artifact, points to consider	Solutions
Is the patient nervous?	Take time to re-explain procedure and relax the patient Use a visualisation technique Use a relaxation technique such as tightening muscles then relaxing them Maintain dignity and keep patient covered
Is the patient gripping the bed or couch sides or are their hands clenched?	Get patient to open hands Raise arms and relax on bed/couch
Is the patient disorientated?	If not crucial to immediate management record later when patient is settled If required immediately or disorientation is long-term distract by chatting through procedure May need assistance
Is the patient shivering from cold?	Record ECGs in a draft free, warm room Cover with a blanket, dressing gown or clothes
Does the patient have Parkinson's disease or other disease associated with myoclonic jerks such as hyperthyroidism?	Choose a time of day when tremor is less marked Tuck the patient's hands under the bottom Place a pillow under the knees Move limb leads further up arms and legs and use a 40Hz filter as a last resort and annotate tracing
Is the patient's body fully supported on the bed or couch?	Ensure patient is comfortable and there is enough room for arms to lie at the patient's side, if not place arms across abdomen
Is the artifact occurring only with inspiration?	Use manual recording mode and record long strips of each lead to ensure 3 consecutive artifact free beats in each lead Bring the original tracing to physician's attention

2. Motion artifact

Motion artifact occurs for several related reasons including:

- the patient moving part of their body
- electrode movement – pressing on the electrode and skin stretching
- vibrations from the environment
- hiccups
- respiratory swing.

Any movement for example when patients move their limbs, fingers, torso or head during an ECG recording produces motion artifact. These body movements also cause muscle tension and therefore EMG artifact. Movement may also loosen the electrode–skin contact strength and/or place tension on the ECG leads. Motion artifact caused by patient movement appears as large baseline shifts up and down the page which may also have an EMG artifact component. The artifact is superimposed on top of the true ECG signal making it difficult to read particularly when it is important to evaluate ST segment changes or measure wave amplitudes (Pyne, 2004).

When the ECG leads pull on the electrodes the skin is stretched (Odman and Oberg, 1982). This may occur if the patient moves as described above or as a result of lead tension. Stretching also occurs when the skin under the electrode is deformed as a result of pressure. Under normal conditions an electrical potential is generated by the ions in the sweat glands and a constant ionic gradient also exists between the inside and outside surfaces of the skin. When the skin is stretched or pressure is put upon it, a piezo-electric effect occurs which converts the stretching or pressure into an electrical potential of several millivolts. The electrical potential generated causes the large baseline shift in the ECG.

Motion artifact may also occur where there are changes in the electrical charge boundary between the electrode–electrolyte interface or the electrolyte–skin interface (Hamilton et al., 2000). Problems between the electrolyte and electrode interface have been greatly reduced with new electrode designs, but the presence of excess sweat, poor skin preparation, body lotions, and poor electrode adhesive quality allow the electrodes to slip, causing changes in the electrical charge at the electrolyte–skin interface.

Another cause of motion artifact is bumping into the patient's bed or couch, the performance of chest compressions, or trying to record in a moving environment such as an ambulance. Vibrations from the environment are passed through the body causing it to move slightly. This is picked up along with the ECG signals.

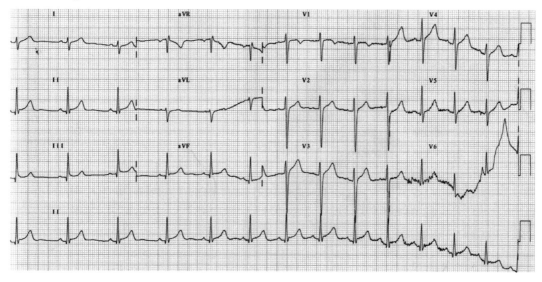

Figure 9.2: Motion artifact caused by patient movement showing characteristic large baseline shifts with an electromyogenic component.

Motion artifact is one of the most common forms of artifact and leads to problems when analysing the ECG. This is because some motion signals are bigger and overlap those of the ECG whilst others are smaller and resemble the true P, Q, R, S and T waves in shape (Thakor and Zhu, 1991). Apart from hiccups and respiratory swing motion artifact described later in this chapter artifact is not regular so cannot be predicted. Due to its unpredictability motion artifact is difficult to remove from the ECG. Digital filters, adaptive noise cancelling and wavelet transform can all help reduce motion artifact but these significantly affect the true ECG waveforms. The use of notch filters during the recording of ECGs is not recommended (AHA, 2007, SCST 2010).

Table 9.2: Steps to limit or remove general motion artifact.

Motion artifact – points to consider	Solutions
Can you see the patient moving?	Ask the patient to lie still and not talk as the recording is made
Can you identify which limb is moving?	If yes make sure the limb is comfortable
Are the mains cable or ECG leads pulling?	Remove tension from the leads
Are the leads suspended and/or swaying?	Reposition leads by placing the lead system on the patient's stomach or close beside them
Is the patient tapping the electrodes or leads intermittently or in a rhythmic fashion?	Reposition leads out of reach of fingers Place hands under the bottom
Are the leads too short to reach without pulling?	Remove any tangles in the leads In tall/obese patients use longer lead sets Use electrodes with offset connectors to absorb tugs on the electrodes and leads
Are you recording whilst moving the patient?	If not clinically detrimental stop momentarily
Is the patient a small child or baby?	Distract with toys, sounds and music Ask the parent or carer to hold the child lying in their arms For babies connect all electrodes and leads then swaddle child firmly in a blanket

Hiccups cause transient changes in intrathoracic pressure and tend to be relatively regular in nature. They make the patient's chest jump and sometimes the limbs tighten in response to the repeated involuntary movement. This causes a roughly regular type of motion artifact in the ECG tracing (Cheng and Miller, 1953). Hiccups can give the impression of premature beats when large in amplitude or extra P waves or U waves when low in amplitude. Where they occur at the same time as an ECG wave the artifact is added to the wave making it larger and/or distorted in shape. Hiccups are particularly common in newborns and infants.

Respiratory swing is commonly seen in patients with chronic obstructive pulmonary disease, or the very nervous hyperventilating patient. The over exaggerated up and down motion of the chest wall moves the electrodes and leads, stretching the skin and causing the artifact. The baseline moves up during inspiration and down during expiration typically at a frequency of around 0.15 to 0.3Hz. The exaggerated motion of the chest wall may also cause changes in the position of the heart and its axis. This can be seen in the ECG as a morphological beat to beat variation usually in QRS height. Respiratory swing can be reduced by using high pass filters or wavelet transform which removes repetitive trends in the ECG baseline.

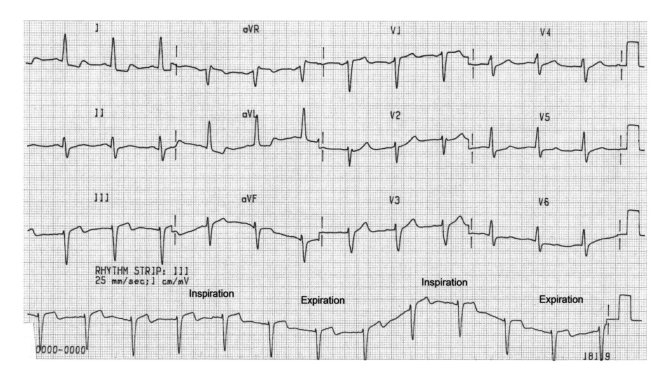

Figure 9.3: Respiratory motion due to deep breathing moving the chest up and down and stretching the skin underneath the electrodes.

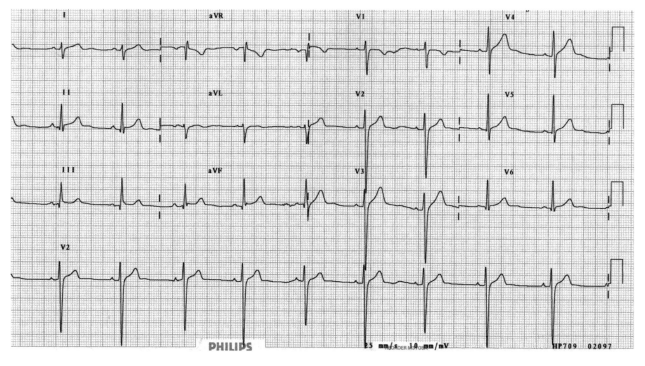

Figure 9.4: Respiratory swing affecting the amplitude of the QRS seen as a beat to beat difference in QRS which is particularly marked in leads V1 and V2.

Table 9.3: Steps to limit or remove hiccups and respiratory swing motion artifact.

Motion artifact – hiccups and respiratory swing, points to consider	Solutions
Can you see/hear the patient hiccupping?	Wait for hiccups to settle Record in manual mode to see how much the ECG can be attained
Is the patient suffering from dyspnoea, breathing very deeply or hyperventilating?	If treatable e.g. an asthmatic attack wait for medication to work then record unless in an emergency In deep breathing ask the patient to inhale and hold breath then record (Almasi and Schmitt, 1974)
Is the artifact associated with orthopnoea?	Prop the patient up to a maximum of 45° angle or record with the patient sitting as a last resort and clearly annotate Record when less breathless or after medication?

3. Poor skin preparation

The outer layer of the skin is composed of dry dead skin cells. This increases the electrical impedance (resistance to electrical flow) reducing the ease with which electrical potentials can pass from the body to the electrodes to be recorded. Impedance is measured in Ohms Ω. Unprepared skin has impedances as high as 100,000–200,000Ω. But a good quality tracing can only be obtained when skin impedance is less than 5,000Ω. To reduce the impedance down to this value the outer layer of the epidermis is removed and then electrolyte is used to improve transfer of the electrical potentials.

The skin also has a large number of sweat glands. Sweat produces electrical potentials as it contains electrically charged ions such as sodium. These interact with the electrolyte of the electrode producing a battery effect where charge can be stored and discharged causing spikes in the ECG. If sweating is excessive and occurs over a large area of the chest a saline bridge forms which in effect causes a short circuit between the electrodes linked by sweat. Excessive sweating also makes the electrodes slip on the skin. Poor skin preparation can appear similar to motion artifact with large swings in the baseline or similar to static electrical artifact/myogenic artifact with spikes. Skin structure and preparation is fully covered in chapter 4.

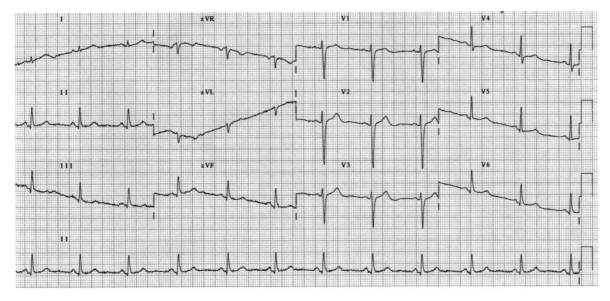

Figure 9.5: Poor skin preparation.

Table 9.4: Steps to limit or remove poor skin preparation artifact.

Poor skin preparation – points to consider	Solutions
Has the skin been adequately prepared following the recommended steps?	Follow the guidelines for preparing skin carefully
Is the patient's skin visibly soiled or does it feel greasy, or has the patient recently used moisturising lotion or other skin care products including topical medications?	Repeat skin preparation and an alcohol based product may be required
Does the patient work with metal?	Very small particles of metal can contaminate skin causing spike artifact. Repeat skin preparation
Is excessive hair present?	Seek consent to remove hair beneath electrode sites
Does the patient have any skin conditions?	Place limb electrodes more medially or laterally Chest electrodes must be on the correct anatomical positions. Omit electrodes affected and annotate reason on ECG
Is the patient visibly sweating or do they feel clammy to the touch?	Reduce room temperature, remove excess clothing and repeat skin preparation

Non-physiological artifact

Non-physiological artifact is predominantly due to electrical artifact which may occur for several reasons including:

- ground loop artifact
- open ECG lead wires, loose electrode–lead connections and loose electrode–skin connections
- offset potential artifact and static electrode popping artifact
- electrical field artifact.

Sustained or intermittent mains electrical artifact is seen in the ECG as a wide, fuzzy baseline of spikes equally spaced and of equal height. When slowed down, 50 spikes or cycles per second (50Hz) may be counted in the UK and 60 per second in the USA (60Hz). Occasionally harmonics of these frequencies are seen (a multiple of 50 or 60Hz). It is very distorting to all parts of the ECG although the QRS peak may still be visible in some leads. Transient electrical artifacts are seen as a large jump or spike in the ECG tracing. In most cases transient electrical artifacts allow the ECG to still be seen clearly for the most part.

1. Ground loop problems

When an electrocardiograph, powered by mains electricity is connected to the patient, the equipment is earthed (grounded) through the earth terminal provided by the mains circuit wiring. When only the electrocardiograph is connected to the patient there should be no electrical artifact assuming the earth system is working correctly and there are no other problems present such as a damaged lead. However, when the patient is also connected to other pieces of mains powered equipment both the electrocardiograph and the other devices all are earthed through the mains network via the sockets. Each socket may have its own earth impedance back to the common earthing point. Electrical artifact arises when there are different earth impedances between each piece of electrical equipment. For example, if an intravenous infusion pump is attached to an earth at higher impedance than the electrocardiograph, then trace electrical current will flow from the infusion pump, through the patient, into the ECG leads, into the electrocardiograph and finally dissipate to ground. The presence of this electrical current will be detected along with the ECG signals.

Ground loop problems have important safety implications if a fault occurs and there are large leakage currents present. Leakage current is the flow of fault current to ground which will then be detected by earth leakage protection equipment in the supply distribution board or in the socket. Electrical devices may leak very small currents to ground and if the leakage current is below the level of the earth leakage protection, these currents will go undetected. However if a fault is present the amount of current leaking to ground may be large. If the situation arises where the patient is connected to two pieces of equipment both separately earthed at different earth impedances, the leakage current will take the path of least impedance to earth. In other words it will flow from the faulty device (assuming this has the higher earth impedance) through the patient and into the ground via the lower earth impedance on another piece of equipment. This may result in an electrical shock if the current flowing is of sufficient magnitude.

Some modern ECG machines do not ground the patient and only the ECG machine is grounded through the power socket. Instead the right leg electrode often referred to as the 'earth or ground lead' connected via an isolation amplifier is used to detect the potential of the patient's body. Any induced AC current (or common mode voltage – an input signal to the amplifier common to two or more leads) flowing in the body is fed to two averaging parallel high 5 Mega Ohm (5M) resistors, inverted, amplified and fed back to the right leg lead. This results in reducing the electrical interference and grounding the patient in another way (Winter and Webster, 1983). This method is called a driven right leg circuit design.

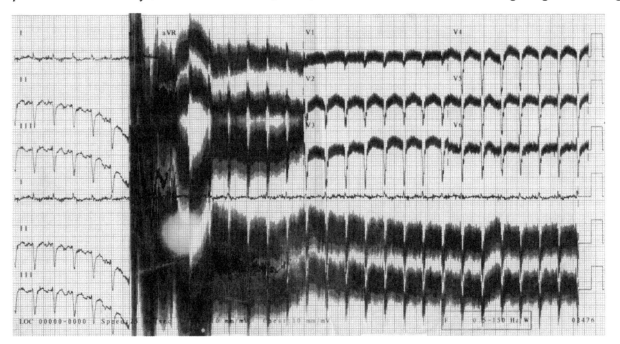

Figure 9.6: Ground loop electrical interference.

2. Open ECG lead wires, loose electrode–lead connections and loose electrode–skin connections

If the ECG lead cables have broken wires internally then open ECG lead artifact may arise. Wires may break when they are roughly handled, excessively stretched, tied in knots or become caught in the ECG machine wheels. In effect this means that the ECG electrode is no longer in good contact with the corresponding ECG lead and acts as an antenna allowing high potentials to be induced in the lead as a result of the surrounding electric fields. Impedance in the lead/s will be high and this feature forms the test for broken leads using an ohmmeter. The same effect as an open lead occurs if the connection between the electrode and the skin is poor or broken.

Sustained or intermittent ground loop, open ECG lead wires, and loose electrode–skin connections may all be reduced by using internal filters in the ECG machine. This type of electrical interference is considered to be narrow band noise, in other words it occurs at 50Hz UK (or 60Hz USA) and has a bandwidth of less than 1Hz. This is very different in frequency to ECG waves and so can be easily removed from the tracing. In most instances the internal filters that meet the recommended standards will remove AC interference without compromising ECG morphology. A notch filter should not be used as this will alter the ECG morphology. Lead integrity should be checked regularly as although filters may improve the recording they do not deal with the underlying cause of the artifact.

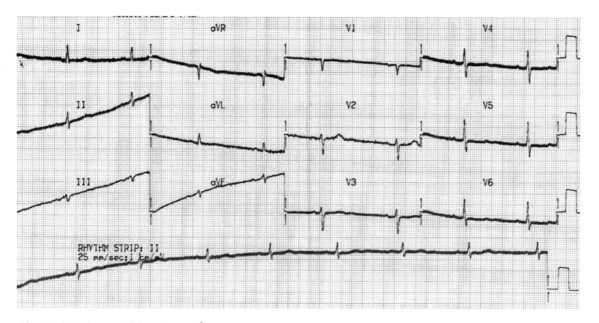

Figure 9.7: Open ECG wire artifact.

Warning

An alternating electrical current which passes from one skin surface electrode through the body may have serious safety hazards. It is the size of the current measured in Milliamps (mA) or Amps (A) that is important rather than the voltage. The severity of the physiological effects increase as the Amps increase from mild tingling to severe burns and death. Examples are shown below for approximate currents which can vary depending upon environmental conditions and the individual affected.

Current	Physiological effect
1mA	a minimum current that can be felt by humans – causes tingling
5mA	the maximal harmless level – between 5 and 8mA pain is felt
8–30mA	involuntary muscular contraction occurs – can't let go
50–150mA	severe muscular reactions and pain, possible respiratory arrest
700+mA	nervous system disruption, ventricular fibrillation, likely to be fatal
6A	sustained cardiac contraction, burns, brain damage, respiratory paralysis

Table 9.5: Steps to limit or remove general electrical artifact.

Ground loop, open wire, loose electrode lead connections and loose skin–electrode artifact, points to consider	Solutions
Is the patient surrounded by mains powered clinical or other equipment?	Turn off all non-essential electrical equipment Run all essential equipment including the electrocardiograph on battery power
Are the mains cables or leads from the ECG machine tangled around other equipment cables and leads?	Separate mains cables and leads
Is the wall socket damaged?	If visibly damaged report and run equipment on battery
Has the electrocardiograph been recently checked for electrical safety?	Regular electrical safety checks are a legal requirement If no evidence of a safety check is available do not use equipment
Are all connections secured?	Check all connections are tight
Are you using a multiple plug adaptor to connect to the mains?	Connect directly to the wall socket, do not use adaptors
Is there any visible damage to the mains cable and/or ECG leads?	Replace damaged ECG lead systems with a spare and return damaged set for repair If spares are not available remove equipment from use and follow department protocol in relation to repair
Is there a good connection between the electrodes and ECG leads?	Check all leads are tightly connected to the electrodes
Are the connections clean and not corroded?	Remove any build-up of electrolyte and replace corroded connectors
Has the skin been properly prepared so that electrodes make close secure contact?	Prepare the skin again and reapply the electrodes If using alcohol to cleanse the skin make sure the skin has dried before applying electrodes
Are the electrodes viable?	Check the electrolyte has not dried out Check the electrodes are within their use by date Check the adhesive properties of the electrode
Other tips to try	Move the ECG machine to the other side of the bed or couch and make sure patient is not touching the metal parts of bed or couch Try turning the ECG machine by 90° Try straightening the ECG leads so they lie parallel with the patient's body

3. Offset potential artifact and static electrode popping

Offset potential artifact is transient and seen as a sudden jump upwards in the ECG. The signal then falls below baseline and slowly drifts back to the baseline where it stabilises. Sometimes the jump is so large that it goes off the page or screen. It is commonly seen on a small scale when electrodes are first applied to the skin. A much larger offset potential is observed briefly after defibrillation when the ECG machine is still recording. The artifact is due to saturation of the amplifiers inside the ECG machine caused by the sudden high step up in the input voltage. This results in the build-up of charge on the coupling capacitors inside the amplifier for a fixed period of time before it discharges and drifts back to its original state. In modern machines the amount of offset due to defibrillation is minimised by using internal electronic protection circuits. This limits the amount of voltage that is allowed to reach the amplifiers and so saturation of the amplifiers is also reduced as is charge build-up. The overall effect is that the shift from baseline is smaller than unprotected internal circuitry and the time to stabilise the baseline is reduced. This is important as after defibrillation it is important to see the ECG rhythm as soon as possible and the ECG machine components are protected from damage.

Older single channel ECG machines also create offset potential artifact when they are manually switched from one lead to another. The artifact occurs because each electrode has a different offset potential. This artifact sometimes occurs with modern multichannel machines when used in manual mode but is reduced when used in automatic mode as during lead switching the offset potentials are discharged and so do not appear on the tracing. When seen in automatic mode it is generally at the start of the tracing and occurs because the electrodes were not given time to stabilise before the recording was made.

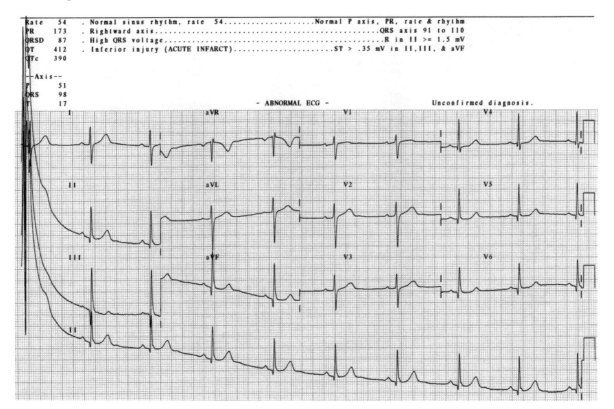

Figure 9.8: Offset potential artifact.

Offset potential is also responsible for static electrode popping. Static electricity originates from synthetic bedding and patient clothing. An electrical charge builds up on these materials and then is discharged through the body to the ECG electrodes. Electrodes are capable of storing the charge. The amount of charge that can be stored and the time it takes for it to discharge and disappear depends upon the electrolyte and the materials the electrode is made from. In general terms, the poorer the ECG electrode, the higher the charge build up and the longer the discharge time, the greater the likelihood of artifact. When the charge stored on the electrodes discharges a single spike, a short burst of spikes, or a small hump is seen in the tracing. Static charge also originates with the practitioner which is then transferred to the patient and into the ECG machine or transferred directly into the ECG machine. The currents associated with static electricity pose no risks. To minimise static electrode popping and to reduce the time for baseline stabilisation following defibrillation silver-silver chloride electrodes are used as they keep offset potentials to a minimum as they do not permit the large build-up of charge.

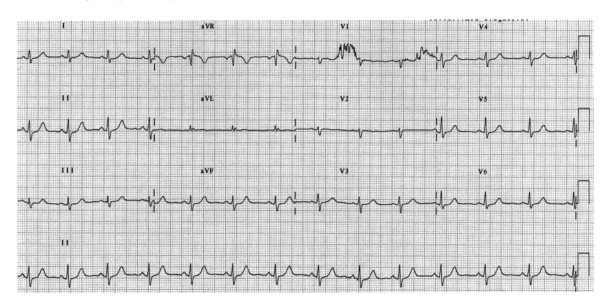

Figure 9.9: Electrode popping artifact caused by static build-up is seen in lead V1.

Table 9.6: Steps to limit or remove offset potential and electrode popping electrical artifact.

Offset potential and electrode popping artifact, points to consider	Solutions
Has the patient just been defibrillated whilst still connected to the ECG machine?	Record on manual during defibrillation so that a longer ECG strip with stable baseline may be obtained to determine rhythm If recording on automatic during defibrillation re-record again once baseline has stabilised
Has the patient just had electrodes applied?	Check baseline is stable before recording If this is a persistent problem check if silver-silver chloride electrodes are being used
Is the ECG machine an old single channel design?	Record longer strips of each lead and use only the sections with stable baselines for interpretation
Is the patient wearing synthetic clothing or bedclothes which have built up charge? Is the ambient humidity less than 40%? Are recording personnel experiencing static build-up?	Try removing materials Ask patient to touch metal part of bed If humidity is low, static electricity can build up Touch the metal part of the bed before the patient – this allows static to discharge through the bed to earth

4. Electric field problems

Clinical areas can be contaminated by electrical artifact from numerous sources including drips, ventilators and personal electronic equipment belonging to the patient. In addition electric cables in the floor, walls and ceiling and the possible close proximity of large electromagnetic fields emanating from another department such as radiography can also result in high levels of electrical artifact being detected. These problems cause electrical artifact in two ways:

- electric field coupling from the power line to the ECG leads or the power line to the patient
- magnetic induction

Electric field coupling occurs when the mains supply, and/or the mains cable between the wall socket and the electrocardiograph come into close proximity with an electrical field. The field interacts with the patient, the ECG leads and the electrocardiograph to create a capacitance or stored charge. The stored charge will either flow to ground through the mains cable and therefore does not cause interference in the ECG. Or it can flow from the mains to an ECG lead and through the electrode into the skin and the patient, from there it creates interference in the ECG before grounding through the patient. Electric field coupling is reduced by using shielded ECG leads where the shield is grounded at the ECG machine. It is also reduced by using common mode rejection filtering in the amplifiers, reducing skin–electrode impedance and raising amplifier input impedance.

Magnetic induction occurs when the current in the power supply creates a magnetic field around the power cable. Magnetic field induction artifact can also occur from nearby fluorescent lights, other pieces of electrical equipment, mobile phones and electrical transformers.

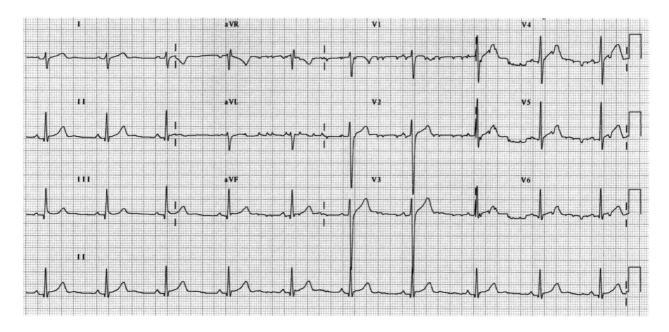

Figure 9.10: Electromagnetic artifact from an analogue mobile phone.

Table 9.7: Steps to limit or remove magnetic induction artifact.

Magnetic induction artifact, points to consider	Solutions
Is there a mobile/cell phone in the vicinity?	Switch phone off
Does the patient have any implanted devices such as nerve stimulators? Does the patient have an old-fashioned FM transmitter/receiver type hearing aid where the receiver box is worn in e.g. a breast pocket of shirt/blouse?	Some nerve stimulators emit signals regularly producing spikes. Nothing can be done in this case Hearing aids may be temporarily switched off
Are you trying to record an ECG where diathermy is being used?	Stop diathermy during recording period
Is the ECG recording room sited next door to the X-ray, MRI or CT department?	Try locating room elsewhere or investigate additional room shielding techniques

5. Electrolyte bridging or gel short-circuit

Electrolyte bridging occurs when too much electrode gel is applied under reusable electrodes such as Welsh suction cup electrodes. The electrolyte runs together forming a short circuit where the signals are picked up and averaged over the larger bridged area. The waveforms recorded will appear the same for all the electrodes joined by the bridge. The use of reusable electrodes is not recommended due to cross infection risks, however if your department has not made this important change then only use a small amount of gel under each electrode, store gel away from heat sources so it remains dense enough not to run but liquid enough to fill crevices in the skin without trapping air (Roy *et al.*, 2007). A similar artifact occurs with modern disposable electrodes when excessive sweating results in bridging or when two or more electrodes are overlapped. With overlapped electrodes the same tracings may be obtained or even artifactual ST elevation produced as signals are composited (Mirvas *et al.*, 1989). By using the correct size of electrode all precordial electrodes can be correctly placed without overlapping even on the smallest adult chest. When applying any monitoring electrodes these should be located away from the standard 12-lead ECG positions. In young children, particularly premature babies, electrode overlapping is a potential problem. Specially designed small paediatric and premature baby ECG electrodes should be used to prevent electrode overlap and ensure anatomical accuracy of electrode placement. If even paediatric ECG electrodes are too large the ECG should be recorded in manual mode, recording alternate precordial electrodes. This will necessitate two recordings to ensure all leads are obtained. The ECG will need to be clearly annotated to ensure there is no confusion in relation to which leads are present on each recording.

6. Saturation or cut-off distortion and printer blocking artifact

When there are high offset potentials at the electrodes, or the amplifiers and filters are inappropriately set then saturation artifact occurs. This is seen in the ECG as squared peaks in the QRS. The sharp narrow peaks cannot be reproduced as the amplifiers cannot exceed their saturation value or the filters have reduced the frequency of waves that can be accurately observed. Printer blocking artifact looks the same as saturation but occurs when the amplitude or height of the cardiac waveforms are greater than the ECG machine's printing space availability or ability. This occurs almost exclusively with the QRS waves. When QRSs are slightly large the equipment will print the waves overlapping making them difficult to separate for interpretation. But if the amplitude is exceptionally large the top of the waveforms are cut-off and appear squared instead of the expected sharp peak. This may be rectified by reducing the gain or amplification to half voltage (5mm/mV) to separate the waveforms and ensure that the points of the QRSs are accurately represented on paper. It is usual only to reduce the leads affected rather than all 12 leads.

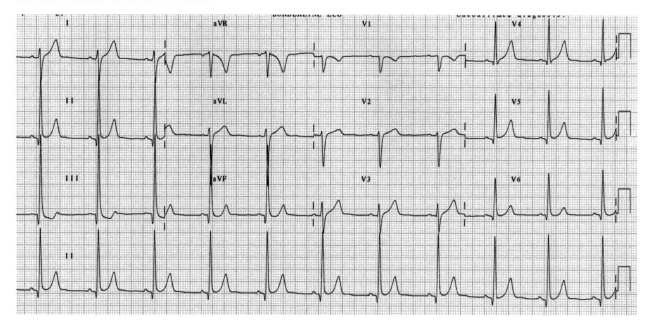

Figure 9.11: Overlapping QRS complexes in I, II, III, aVL and aVF.

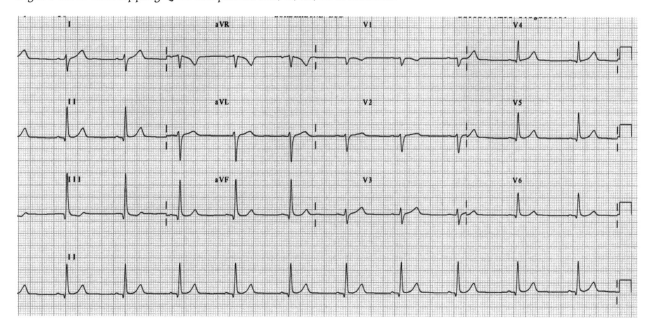

Figure 9.12: ECG from figure 9.11 recorded at half voltage; note the calibration marker has changed to 5mm high indicating the tracing was recorded at a sensitivity of 0.5mV = 10mm.

7. Intermittent or no tracing

Breaks in any part of the patient cable or loose connections can cause intermittent loss of the ECG or no tracing at all. A broken lead or loose connection may be identified by the lead or set of leads affected in the ECG. For instance, a broken or damaged left arm lead will affect lead I and lead III, but not lead II. In some electrocardiographs if a limb lead is broken no tracing will be recorded in any lead the electrode provides a potential for. For example if the left arm lead is broken, the ECG will show only lead II. No tracing will be seen in any of the augmented leads or the precordial leads.

100

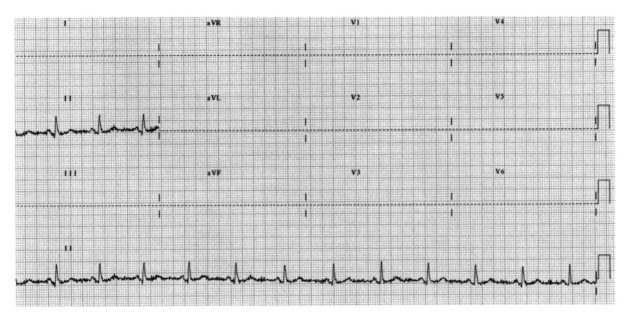

Figure 9.13: Broken left arm lead.

A missing or intermittent tracing in a single precordial lead will be due to that lead alone for example V1 in figure 9.14. Another source of no tracing is the use of different electrodes. All electrode brands have different offset potentials and mixing them results in different signal strengths. Where different metals or compositions are used a poor quality signal is obtained or in some cases no signal at all.

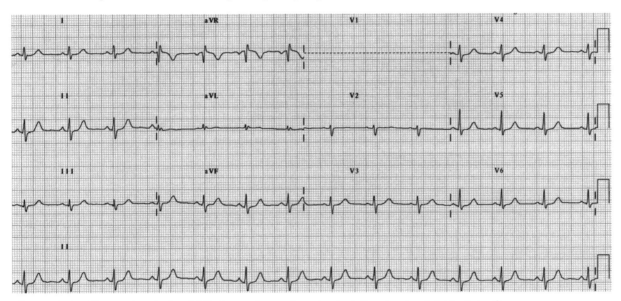

Figure 9.14: No tracing in lead V1 due to loss of contact at the electrode/skin interface.

Table 9.8: Steps to limit or remove intermittent or no tracing artifact.

Intermittent or no tracing artifact, points to consider	Solutions
Are the lead connections tight?	Loose connections may result in no tracing, intermittent tracings or tracings which resemble coarse ventricular fibrillation. Check all connections are tight
Are electrodes all the same brand and type and are not dried up?	Use viable electrodes Do not mix brands

cont.

Are electrodes secured well on skin?	Check that good contact has been achieved
Are you using connectors and tab electrodes?	Check clips the right way round; the metal plate must be in contact with the metal underside of the tab electrode
Are you certain of the lead integrity?	Replace cable Have leads checked
Are you using thermal printing paper?	Check the paper is correctly loaded; some thermal papers will print on one side only

8. Lead reversal

Reversing the ECG leads accidently can cause changes that mimic pathological conditions. The left arm, left leg and right arm of electrodes can be misplaced in five different combinations, when the right leg earth electrode is added this increases the misplacement possibilities up to eighteen different combinations. With four limb leads and six chest leads the possible number of reversal combinations has been calculated at more than three and a half million (Schijvenaars *et al.*, 2008). The possibility of making a mistake is high. The most common reversals are between two limb leads or two chest leads. It is rarer to swap a chest and limb lead as they are of different size and so the fault is more obvious. However the likelihood of this fault occurring is increased in leads of the same colour and/or when leads have been replaced with a non-labelled substitute.

Limb lead reversal

In theory, reversing the limb leads should never happen as there is both an ECG colour code sequence to be followed and modern ECG interpretive programs warn of some lead reversals. However when attention is not paid to the recording technique or the subsequent tracing obtained errors may still occur. Lead reversal can be difficult to spot in some arrhythmias or if the right and left legs have been swapped. Limb lead reversal can be collateral i.e. the arm leads are swapped with each other or the leg leads are swapped with each other. Reversal can also be homolateral i.e. an arm lead is swapped with a leg lead. The table below describes the changes expected when limb lead reversal occurs in sinus rhythm. It can be clearly seen that mixing up the limb leads affects the ECG report given, however only one combination (right arm left arm reversal) produced a warning (see figures 9.15–9.18).

Table 9.9: Steps to remove limb lead reversal artifact.

Limb lead reversal artifact, points to consider	Solutions
Is the P wave amplitude greater in lead I than in lead II? i.e. there has been a shift in P wave axis to the left	Left arm and left leg have been reversed (Abdollah and Milliken, 1997) – check and re-record ECG with correct limb connections
Has the P wave in lead III got an unexpected positive terminal component? i.e. is biphasic	Can be difficult to spot unless a previous ECG is available
Does aVR appear to be unaffected compared to the other limb leads? Is the patient in atrial flutter?	If the saw toothed F waves are clearly visible in leads I, III and aVL but not II – then likely to be left arm left leg lead reversal (Abdollah and Milliken, 1997)
Does the patient have acute coronary syndrome with known ST elevation in inferior leads?	If conflicting evidence visible in the ECG such as ST elevation in leads I and aVL, with possible depression in III and aVF – then left arm left leg lead reversal should be suspected (Akel *et al.*, 2004)

Is the P wave negative in lead I and aVL? Is P wave and R wave positive in aVR? Is there extreme axis deviation of +180° to -90° present? Is R wave negative in lead I and positive in aVF?	Right arm and left arm have been reversed; check and re-record ECG with correct limb connections Check patient does not have dextrocardia i.e. if patient is still available re-record ECG being very careful with lead connections; if patient is unavailable and there is no X-ray or documented evidence of dextrocardia look for primarily negative complexes in leads V3 to V6. The T waves in V3 to V6 may or may not be inverted, this depends on underlying pathology
Is lead II very flat looking <0.1mV in amplitude? Is lead III upside down? Does aVR and aVF look very similar?	If lead II is low voltage right leg and right arm may have been reversed. Voltage is low because there is practically no difference in voltage between the right arm electrode misplaced on the right leg and the left leg voltages. (Usually the right leg voltage is not measured but acts as an earth.) If lead III is low voltage right leg and left arm have been reversed Check and re-record ECG with correct limb connections
Does the ECG resemble an inferior myocardial infarction? Does aVF look like what would be expected in aVR? Is the P wave inverted in aVF?	It is likely in the absence of evidence for a true inferior myocardial infarction that the right arm and left leg leads have been reversed

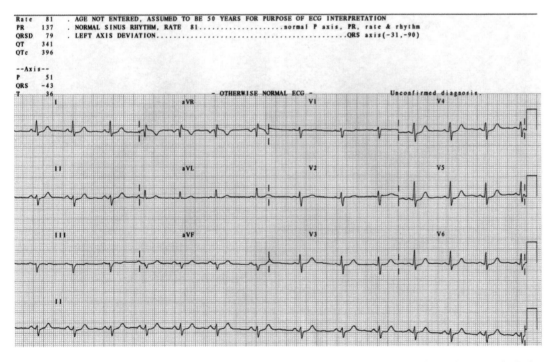

Figure 9.15: Tracing with all electrodes placed in the standardised limb and precordial electrode positions.

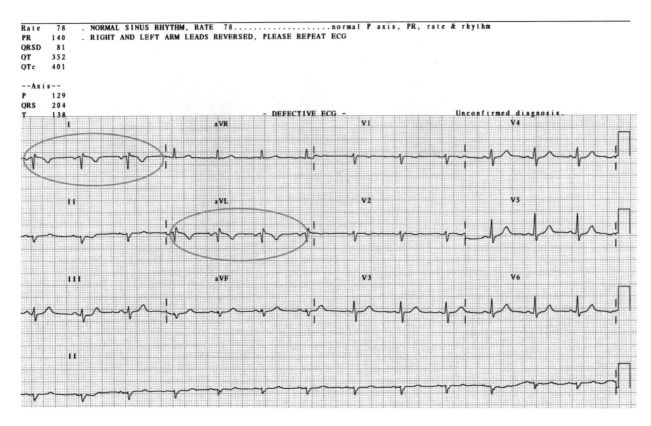

Figure 9.16: Tracing of right and left arm lead reversal also called technical dextrocardia. The computerised ECG report has recognised this common mistake and asked for the ECG to be repeated.

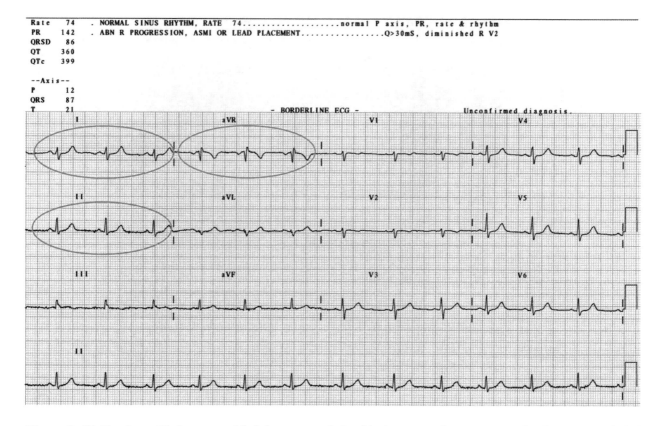

Figure 9.17: Tracing of left arm and left leg reversal. In this instance the P wave in lead I is very slightly larger than that in V2. Lead aVR looks exactly like the normal aVR tracing in figure 9.15.

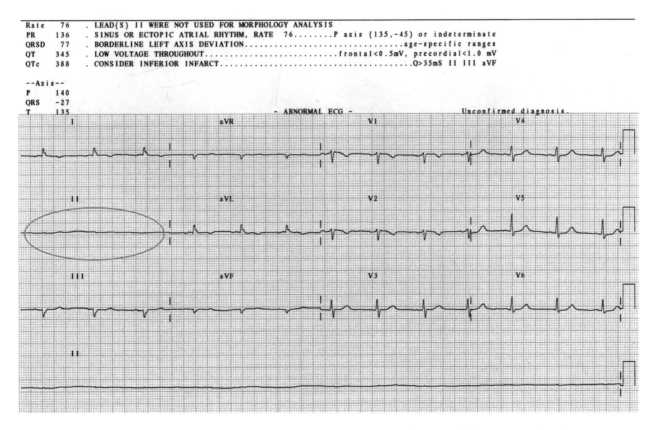

```
Rate    76    . LEAD(S) II WERE NOT USED FOR MORPHOLOGY ANALYSIS
PR     136    . SINUS OR ECTOPIC ATRIAL RHYTHM, RATE  76........P axis (135,-45) or indeterminate
QRSD    77    . BORDERLINE LEFT AXIS DEVIATION.................................age-specific ranges
QT     345    . LOW VOLTAGE THROUGHOUT...........................frontal<0.5mV, precordial<1.0 mV
QTc    388    . CONSIDER INFERIOR INFARCT.....................................Q>35mS II III aVF

--Axis--
P      140
QRS    -27
T      135                                - ABNORMAL ECG -                Unconfirmed diagnosis.
```

Figure 9.18: Tracing of right arm and right leg reversal. Lead II is abnormally low in amplitude.

Precordial lead reversal

Currently ECG machines do not provide a warning that the precordial leads have been swapped just as the incorrect placement of the precordial electrodes cannot be recognised. The most common errors are swapping two adjacent leads such as V1 and V2, V2 and V3 and so on. V1 and V6 lead reversal does occur but is relatively easy to spot in the ECG. This error may also occur if leads are not inserted in the correct order into the ECG yoke.

Table 9.10: Steps to remove precordial lead reversal artifact.

Precordial lead reversal, points to consider	Solutions
Is R larger in V1 than V6? Is S wave smaller in V1 than V6?	Reversal of V1 and V6 leads; check and re-record ECG with correct limb connections

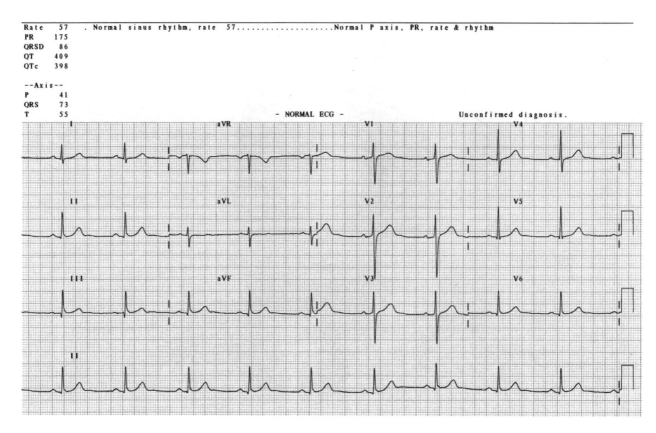

Figure 9.19: Tracing with all electrodes placed in the standardised limb and precordial electrode positions.

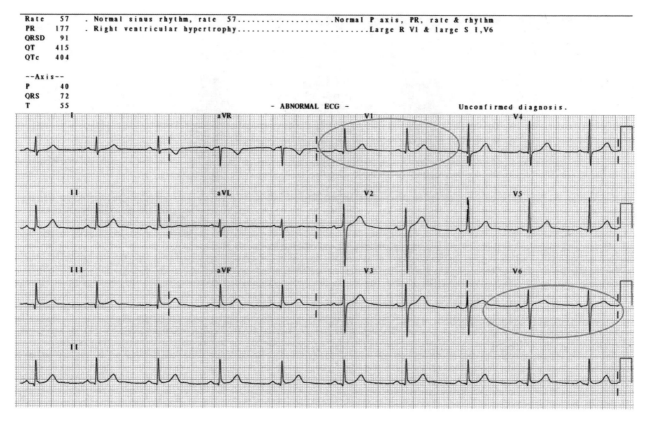

Figure 9.20: V1 and V6 reversal. In this case the artifactual tall R wave in V1 and deep S wave in V6 caused by reversing the electrodes has been reported as right ventricular hypertrophy.

9. Incorrect electrode positioning

This artifact is extremely hard to detect unless the electrode positions are viewed during recording and noted to be incorrect. Once a tracing has been obtained and the electrodes removed there is no way of knowing exactly where electrodes have been placed. The only clues available are new changes that do not make clinical sense or that there is no other supporting evidence for. For example placing the V1 and V2 electrodes too high may produce an ECG with apparent atrial enlargement but a subsequent echocardiogram and other clinical tests and history will not concur. When incorrect electrode placement is suspected another ECG should be recorded and compared as soon as possible. Correct electrode positioning is discussed in chapter 3.

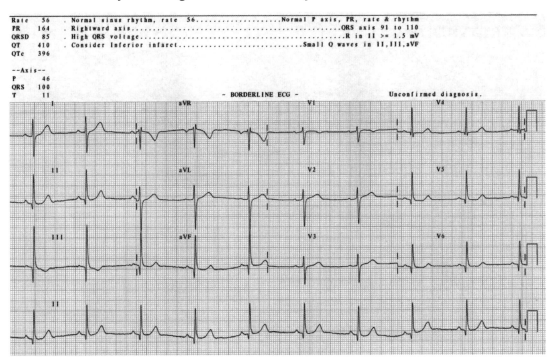

Figure 9.21: Tracing with limb electrodes on tops of arms and legs in same individual as figure 9.19.

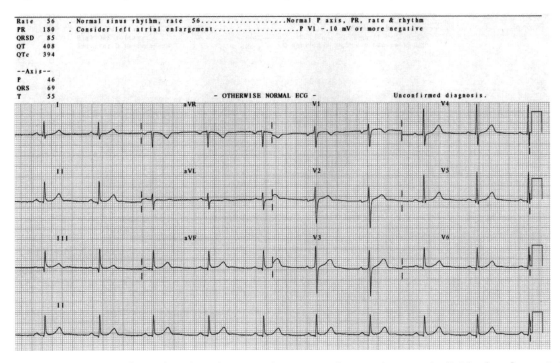

Figure 9.22: V1 and V2 placed in the second intercostal space in same individual as figure 9.19.

Summary of key points:

- Artifact is both unwanted non-cardiac signals and practitioner introduced faults in the ECG. Artifact makes the ECG difficult or impossible to analyse and can lead to misinterpretation and mismanagement.

- There is a wide range of artifacts, each has its own characteristic patterns which allows them to be recognised and appropriate action taken to eliminate or reduce them.

- The practitioner will recognise that both environmental and practitioner factors can result in artifact.

Key review questions

1. If current was accidentally passing through your patient, why might they report a tingling sensation at values less than 1mA?

2. What possible misinterpretation could be made in relation to the ECG in figure 9.11?

3. If the leads attached to the V1 and V2 electrodes were accidently reversed what would you expect to see in the ECG?

References

Abdollah, H., Milliken, J. (1997). 'Recognition of electrocardiographic left arm/left leg lead reversal.' *American Journal of Cardiology*. **80**(9): 1247–49.

Akel R., Saeed, M., Ware, D.L., Chamoun, A.J., Birnbaum, Y. (2004). 'Unusual evolution of ST elevation acute myocardial infarction.' *Annals of Noninvasive Electrocardiology*. **9**(4): 410–14.

Almasi, J.J., Schmitt, O.H. (1974). 'Basic technology of voluntary cardiorespiratory synchronization in electrocardiology.' *Institute of Electrical and Electronics Engineers Transactions on Biomedical Engineering*. **21**: 264–73.

American College Cardiology/American Heart Association. (2001). 'Clinical competence statement on electrocardiography and ambulatory electrocardiography.' *Circulation*. **104**(25): 3169–78.

American Heart Association, American College of Cardiology Foundation, and the Heart Rhythm Society (2007) 'Recommendations for the standardization and interpretation of the electrocardiogram Part I: The electrocardiogram and its technology.' *Journal of the American College of Cardiology* **49**(10): 1128–35.

Bailey, J.J., Berson, A.S., Garson, A., Horan, L.G., Macfarlane, P.W., Mortara, D.W., Zywietz, C. (1990). 'Recommendations for standardisation and specifications in automated electrocardiography: bandwidth and digital signal processing.' *Circulation*. **81**(20):730–39.

Bhatia, L., Turner, D. (2005). 'Parkinson's tremor mimicking ventricular tachycardia.' *Age and Ageing*. **34**: 410–11.

Chase, C., Brady, W.J. (2000). 'Artifactual electrocardiographic change mimicking clinical abnormality on the ECG.' *American Journal of Emergency Medicine*. **18**(3): 312–16.

Cheng, T.O., Miller, A.J. (1953). 'The effect of hiccup on the electrocardiogram: Registration of diaphragmatic action currents and mechanical artifacts.' *American Heart Journal*. **46**: 616–20.

Hamilton, P.S., Curley, M., Roberto, A. (2000). 'Effect of adaptive motion artifact reduction on QRS detection.' *Biomedical Instrumentation and Technology*. **34**(3): 197–202.

Hwang, W.J. (2008). 'Tremor-induced electrocardiographic artifact mimicking atrial flutter.' *Acta Neurologica Taiwanica* **17**(2): 151–2.

Knight, B.P., Pelosi, F., Michaud. G.F., Strickberger, S.A., Moraday, F. (1999) 'Clinical consequences of electrocardiographic artifact mimicking ventricular tachycardia.' *New England Journal of Medicine*. **341**(17): 1270–74.

Knight, B.P., Pelosi, F., Michaud. G.F., Strickberger, S.A., Moraday, F. (2001) 'Physician interpretation of electrocardiographic artifact that mimics ventricular tachycardia.' *The American Journal of Medicine*. **110**(5):335–38.

Littmann, L., Rennyson, S.L., Wall, B.P., Parker, J.M. (2008). 'Significance of respiratory artifact in the electrocardiogram.' *The American Journal of Cardiology*. **102**(8): 1090–96.

Mirvis, D.M., Berson, A.S., Goldberger, A.L., Green, L.S., Heger, J.J., Hinohara, T., Insel, J., Krucoff, M.W., Moncrief, A., Selvester, R.H. (1989). 'Instrumentation and practice standards for electrocardiographic monitoring in special care units. A Report for Health Professionals by a Task Force of the Council on Clinical Cardiology, American Heart Association.' *Circulation*. **79**(2): 464–71.

Odman, S., Oberg, P. (1982). 'Movement induced potentials in surface electrodes.' *Medical and Biological Engineering and Computing*. **20**(2): 159–66.

Pyne, C.C. (2004). 'Classification of acute coronary syndromes using the 12-lead electrocardiogram as a guide.' *American Association of Critical Care Nurses Clinical Issues*. **15**(4): 558–67.

Roy, S.H., De Luca, G., Cheng, M.S., Johansson, A., Gilmore, L.D., De Luca, C.J. (2007). 'Electro-mechanical stability of surface EMG sensors.' *Medical and Biological Engineering and Computing*. **45**(5): 447–57.

Salerno, S.M., Alguire, P.C., Waxman, H.S. (2003). 'Competency in interpretation of 12-lead electrocardiograms: a summary and appraisal of published evidence.' *Annals of Internal Medicine*. **138**(9): 751–60.

Schijvenaars, B.J.A., van Herpen, G., Kors, J.A. (2008). 'Intraindividual variability in electrocardiograms.' *Journal of Electrocardiology*. **41**(3): 190–96.

Smith, M, (1984), 'Rx for ECG monitoring artifact.' *Critical Care Nurse*. **4**(1): 64–6.

Society of Cardiological Science and Technology (2010) 'Clinical Guidelines by Consensus: Recording a standard 12-lead ECG: An Approved Methodology.' Available from: http://www.scst.org.uk/resources/consensus_guideline_for_recording_a_12_lead_ecg_Rev_072010b.pdf (Accessed 6/3/12).

Srikureja, W., Darbar, D., Reeder, G.S. (2000). 'Tremor induced ECG artifact mimicking ventricular tachycardia.' *Circulation*. **102**(11): 1337–38.

Thakor, N.V., Zhu, Y. (1991). 'Applications of adaptive filtering to ECG analysis: noise cancellation and arrhythmia detection.' *Institute of Electrical and Electronics Engineers Transactions on Biomedical Engineering*. **38**(8): 785–94.

Vereckei, A. (2004). 'Pseudo-ventricular tachycardia: electrocardiographic artefact mimicking non-sustained polymorphic ventricular tachycardia in a patient evaluated for syncope.' *Heart* **90**(1): 81.

Winter, B.B., Webster, J.G. (1983). 'Driven right leg circuit design.' *Institute of Electrical and Electronics Engineers Transactions on Biomedical Engineering*. **30**: 62–6.

Chapter 10
The computer generated report

By the end of this chapter you should be able to:
- recognise that computerised reports are not infallible and are not intended to replace the opinion of the practitioner
- appreciate that in artifact free ECG tracings the computer is more accurate at making heart rate, axis and interval measurements than even clinical experts
- understand that the quality of the computer generated report is dependent upon the sophistication of the algorithm used to interpret the data
- evaluate how the quality of electrocardiograph recording affects the computer generated report.

Computerised ECG reporting

Computerised ECG interpretation started in the early 1960s and established electrocardiography as one of the first uses of computers in the healthcare setting. ECG analysis is now routinely incorporated into electrocardiograms and most machines employed in clinical practice have this capability. Computerised analysis systems rely upon two key principles:

- the quality and accuracy of the information recorded. (Data must be artifact free and have been recorded from the standardised anatomical positions.)
- the analysis program's sophistication and interpretative accuracy.

If either of these principles are not met the computerised ECG report will be inaccurate.

Modern computer analysis is excellent at recognising the normal ECG, calculating accurate heart rates, cardiac axis, intervals and voltages in artifact free tracings. It is not good at evaluating the above in noisy tracings nor is it good at interpreting abnormal tracings when multiple and complex abnormalities are present. Frequently normal variants are analysed as abnormal, pacemaker activity is missed and few systems can deal well with paediatric analysis. As yet computer analysis systems cannot correlate a patient's clinical symptoms and history with the ECG data to make a more specific report. Overall studies have shown that the computer analysis cannot substitute for expert interpretation (Sekiguchi *et al.*, 1999). In general a tracing reported as normal may usually be relied upon but one that states or suggests a particular abnormality cannot without further checking.

Computer interpretation is a beneficial tool for the practitioner experienced in ECG interpretation. However it offers little additional benefit to those who are inexperienced or unable to interpret ECGs. Relying on a computerised report without the ability to check its validity may even prove dangerous.

For the experienced ECG interpreter a computerised report:

- provides a second opinion
- may sometimes highlight information that has been overlooked in an emergency situation
- may suggest additional findings to consider
- saves time in physically writing the report as the practitioner can agree or alter the computer report and sign it off. The time is saved in the calculation and measurement part rather than on producing an interpretation based on clinical findings.

Clinical tip

Always make a final scan of the ECG in case anything has been missed by both the healthcare practitioner and the computer. Don't assume this will never happen – it does.

For the inexperienced ECG interpreter a computerised report:

- can be reassuring if the result is reported as normal
- can cause anxiety to both the interpreter and the patient if it is suggestive of an abnormal finding that cannot be immediately confirmed
- may result in inappropriate treatment if diagnosis and management is based on the computerised report
- discourages the need to learn interpretation as too much reliance is inappropriately placed on the accuracy of the computerised report
- encourages the use of learning from the computer rather than critically evaluating the validity of the computer report.

The report produced will only ever be as good as the data it analyses. When the incorrect electrode positions have been used the computerised report is known to produce a clinically significant change in up to 50 per cent of cases (Hill & Goodman, 1987). Even in the most modern equipment only some limb lead reversal mistakes can be recognised. The computer is unable to detect where the limb electrodes or the precordial electrodes have been placed.

Clinical tip

Better interpretation skills are developed by covering the computerised ECG report and writing a report first. This can then be checked against the computer report. Anything that doesn't match should be checked with a more experienced member of staff – don't assume the computer is always correct.

Unstable interpretations

Identical ECG signals will result in identical interpretations and measurements when analysed by the same program. However, even small insignificant signal changes can result in an entirely different computerised interpretation. This is multiplied in the presence of artifact. Unstable interpretations are a particular problem when recording serial ECGs. Tracings recorded only a couple of minutes apart often create completely different reports.

Analysis on different equipment

Equipment from different manufacturers uses different algorithms. Algorithms are sets of rules that have been designed and tested to lead to one conclusion or several closely related conclusions. They are based upon diagnostic criteria and vary between manufacturers. This means that the same patient with exactly the same electrodes in place could produce different ECG reports when two electrocardiographs from different manufacturers are used. Experimentally this has been confirmed by feeding the same raw ECG data into different machines (Salerno *et al.*, 2003). There is a move to standardise the algorithm definitions used by different manufacturers but this has not yet been achieved (AHA, 2007; AHA, 2009).

At the clinic

Working with a colleague, record each other's ECG when relaxed and with muscles tensed. Compare the computerised report for both recordings. Note changes in measurements, rhythm interpretation and overall conclusion.

Overview of the analysis process

ECG analysis programs measure waveform morphologies, durations and amplitudes. The ECG algorithms used are highly specific to patient age and gender. The majority of analysis programs are designed for adult use only however special paediatric interpretation packages can be added. In general the analysis of ECGs takes place in seven main steps:

- Patient demographics used to aid interpretation is entered.
- Standardised electrode positions and lead attachment must be used as analysis algorithms are based upon these.
- All twelve leads of the ECG are acquired simultaneously.
- Each lead is examined for technical quality.
- The waveform components are identified.
- Each component is measured.
- The algorithm is applied to the measurements based on the patient demographic information to select representative pre-set interpretative statements.

Waveform recognition and measurements

In each of the twelve ECG leads recorded the beats are detected and the waveforms are recognised and measured. The shape, amplitude, duration and area under the waves will be calculated for each component of the ECG (P, QRS, ST segment and T). The morphology parameters of the beats are then grouped together. The rate and the morphology parameters establish how the beats are subsequently classified. The presence of each waveform is counted and their relationships to the other waveforms recorded in order to analyse the rhythm present. Measurements are calculated from the most frequently occurring beats. Atrial rhythm parameters are calculated by identifying the number of P waves per QRS complex. Axis measurements are made using the waveform areas. These measurements have a greater accuracy than those calculated manually and this is where computer analysis systems excel.

113

1. Heart rate detection

With beat detection R–R intervals are used to determine if the heart rate is normal (60–100 bpm) in the adult, bradycardic (60 bpm) or tachycardic (100 bpm). Heart rate analysis is important in the computerised reporting process of an ECG.

2. Rhythm classification

Classification systems are used by the computer of the electrocardiograph to decide if the patient is normal or abnormal. If abnormal the computer can compare features and place the ECG into a number of disease states. The classifiers use chains of decision logic algorithms based on probability to determine rhythm based on the statistics collected. For instance if R–R interval ≥ 100bpm then tachycardia is reported. Because swapping some limb leads produces such characteristic changes (table 9.9, page 102) it is possible to use an algorithm to alert the user to check for this. The main difficulty with classification system logic is that it does not deal well with artifact in the tracing and tries to interpret it as a true physiological finding.

The data from the waveform analysis and the R–R intervals together help identify what rhythm and if relevant what arrhythmias are present. Atrial or junctional premature complexes are recognised when the preceding R–R interval is shorter (typically by 15 per cent or more) than the recognised normal R–R interval in the presence of a normal QRS duration. Those with a longer than measured normal QRS duration are classed as being either aberrant supraventricular or ventricular beats. Pauses are categorised by the R–R interval measuring 40 per cent more than the average R–R interval. First degree atrioventricular block is detected by a prolonged PR interval. Second degree atrioventricular block is recognised by having more P waves than QRS complexes. Wenckebach is indicated by progressively longer PR intervals preceding a long R–R interval.

When the QRS duration is prolonged the depolarisation does not arise from the AV node and bundle of His. If the rate is over 100 bpm the computer decision tree logic reports it as a ventricular tachycardia or supraventricular tachycardia. To improve the correct identification of the type of tachycardia present, a Bayesian classifier may be applied. For example in the ventricular case a large sample of R wave amplitude and QRS duration is measured in normal subjects and from subjects in ventricular tachycardia and plotted on a graph of peak voltage against QRS duration. The mean and standard deviation of each group is calculated, and a decision boundary constructed so that if an individual with an unknown rhythm was plotted on the graph the position of the data would indicate what rhythm was present and minimise the probability of making a classification error.

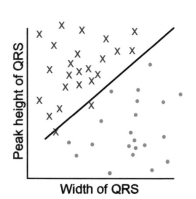

Figure 10.1: Example of a simple Bayesian classifier. X denotes normal sinus rhythm and the dots denote ventricular tachycardia (VT). In the above example no VT is misclassified as sinus but two sinus individuals have been misclassified as VT.

The presence of extra R or S waves in the QRS coupled with prolongation of the QRS duration is reported as a conduction block. Depending on the exact pattern seen it is reported as either a blockage in the left or right bundles or a fascicular block. When the R waves fall below the QRS detection threshold and no waveforms can be identified this is reported as ventricular fibrillation. Similarly the low voltage P waves or absence of P waves can be used to trigger the computer decision tree logic to report atrial fibrillation or atrial tachycardia.

3. Ischaemic heart disease detection

Ischaemic heart disease is detected and classified on the basis of ST segment depression which will be a negative value. The slope of the ST segment and the shape are also considered. The location of the ischaemia can also be indicated from the leads in which it is identified. If the heart rate is rapid (190 minus age in years) the pre-set interpretative statement will normally identify a rate related ST depression.

Summary of key points:

- Computer generated reports are excellent at making measurements and recognising the normal ECG patterns in good quality data. However they cannot as yet replace the critical thinking processes of a skilled healthcare practitioner in establishing the presence of abnormalities particularly when signals are poor.

- The analysis program averages measurements over several beats and calculates axis from the area under the waves. As the signal is digitised for analysis the computer is able to determine minute changes not visible to the naked eye.

- Sophisticated ECG algorithms can support the analysis of data. With the recommended standardisation of algorithms, the analysis of waveforms and rhythms will be more consistent between different manufacturers.

- The accuracy of the report is based on high quality ECG signals being acquired from all electrodes.

Key review questions

1. Why is simultaneous data collection required for computer generated analysis?

2. In relation to the sampling frequency required for digitisation, what is the primary benefit of oversampling?

3. Why might two electrocardiographs with identical diagnostic algorithms produce different reports for the same input?

References

AHA (2007). 'Recommendations for the standardization and interpretation of the Electrocardiogram, Part II: Electrocardiography Diagnostic Statement List: a scientific statement from the American Heart Association Electrocardiography and Arrhythmias Committee, Council on Clinical Cardiology; the American College of Cardiology Foundation and the Heart Rhythm Society.' *Journal of the American College of Cardiology.* **49**: 1128–35

AHA (2009). 'Recommendations for the standardization and interpretation of the electrocardiogram, Part VI: Acute Ischemia/Infarction: a scientific statement from the American Heart Association Electrocardiography and Arrythmias Committee, Council on Clinical Cardiology: the American College of Cardiology Foundation and the Heart Rhythm Association.' *Circulation* 100: e262–e70.

Hill, N.E., Goodman, J. (1987) 'Importance of accurate placement of precordial leads in the 12-lead electrocardiogram.' *Heart & Lung* **16**: 561–6.

Salerno, S.M., Alguire, P.C., Waxman, H.S. (2003). 'Competency in interpretation of 12-lead electrocardiograms: a summary and appraisal of published evidence.' *Annals of Internal Medicine.* **138**(9): 751–60.

Sekiguchi, K., Kanda, T., Osada, M., Tsunoda, Y., Kodajima, N., Fukumura, Y., Suzuki, T., Kobayashi, I. (1999). 'Comparative accuracy of automated computer analysis versus physicians in training in the interpretation of electrocardiograms.' *Journal of Medicine.* **30**(1–2): 75–81.

Chapter 11
Archiving records

By the end of this chapter you should be able to:
- discuss the advantages and disadvantages of different writing systems used for obtaining hardcopy ECGs
- appreciate the role of digital archiving
- appreciate how ECG voltage signals are converted into digital codes for archiving
- understand different methods of transmitting ECG data.

ECGs recorded in the clinical environment must be stored in the department where the ECG has been recorded for three to five years depending on local protocols. The original hardcopies in patient notes are archived again according to local protocol. However in some clinical trials ECGs must be held for up to 15 years. This has proved problematic in hardcopy form, i.e. a paper copy of the ECG, as the process is both space consuming and time consuming as ECGs must be filed alphabetically or by patient number etc. The relatively recent move to digitisation has revolutionised ECG storage, thousands can be stored on hard drives and on external storage devices and management systems. ECGs can also now be transmitted from the recording point to anywhere in the world and stored on central clinical databases along with other investigations such as X-rays, blood results and further patient information.

Archiving Hardcopy ECGs

It is still normal clinical practice to print an ECG on paper. This is then filed with any report or comments into the patient's records, a second hardcopy may be held in the recording department. But there are a number of problems with archiving hardcopy ECGs apart from needing storage space.

- **Reduction of print quality with time** – some ECG papers particularly those recorded on thermal paper either fade in time or become blackened in exposure to light or heat sources. This can be overcome by making a high quality photocopy and storing with the original ECG. The ECG gridlines should be clearly visible on the photocopy so that voltage and timing measurements can still be calculated. The ECG should also be photocopied straight and not running at an angle up the page.

- **Disposal of hardcopies** – at some point in time the ECGs can be destroyed. As the ECGs contain confidential details and information they must be destroyed following the local confidential waste protocol.

- **Misfiling and loss** – ECGs can be misfiled or mislaid and therefore a second copy is not always available despite best intentions. It is also time consuming to file and access the ECGs.

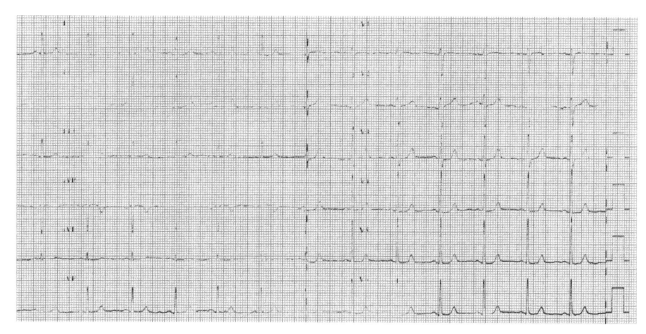

Figure 11.1: Faded ECG tracing.

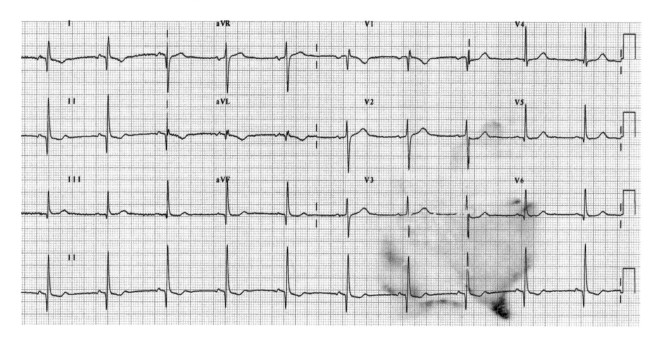

Figure 11.2: Light heat damage to ECG tracing seen as the blackened area on the lower right.

The storage of hardcopy ECGs will depend upon the paper they have been recorded on or the method used to create the tracing on the paper.

Thermal activated paper

Thermal ECG paper is activated to leave a tracing when it comes in contact with a heated stylus or a thermal print head such as a thermal array dot printer. ECGs printed on thermal paper are not suitable for long-term storage. Even when carefully stored they only have a lifespan of three to five years at most before they start to fade. Factors that may help to prolong the life of the original tracing:

- store inside paper envelopes to keep out light (avoid self-adhesive foils used for some filing systems)

- keep away from heat, visible light, neon and ultraviolet light sources e.g. don't store close to a radiator or in front of a sunny window or neon signs
- accidental exposure to cleaning fluids such as alcohol wipes and ether will affect the tracing
- do not use alcohol or ether based glues if sticking onto a surface
- handle at the edges of the tracing as warm, greasy fingers can leave marks
- do not rub, scratch or fold the paper as friction leaves marks
- do not store in PVC plastic pockets as some papers interact and turn black
- a high quality photocopy should be made
- thermal paper should be stored below 27.8 degrees Centigrade or 80 degrees Fahrenheit
- humidity should not exceed 65 per cent.

Ink jet or laser printed ECGs:

- can be stored directly filed into charts or inside plastic pockets or envelopes
- no special storage is required.

Single channel strip recorders

Some old types of ECG machine print only one lead at a time. The resulting ECG is a very long strip of paper. This type of format is difficult to store due to its bulk when folded. The ECG therefore needs to be mounted or stored wound around card. To mount the ECG short strips of each lead are cut to show three to five complexes depending on heart rate. These are labelled and stuck onto card in order of the normal 12-lead ECG sequence. An alternative is to wind the ECGs around card. One end of the ECG is glued onto the card then the ECG is wrapped around and the free end secured in place with a paperclip.

Archiving Digitised ECGs or paperless storage

Many biological signals including the ECG are described as electrical analogue signals. In the case of the ECG the voltages measured vary over time to create waveforms of varying amplitude. For computers to be able to analyse the waveforms the voltages or amplitudes must be sampled regularly and the measurements made converted into a series of numbers. A single ECG complex would be sampled several hundred times, each sample producing a number. This is achieved through an analogue to digital converter. For the conversion to be accurate the number of samples taken must be very high or else information between the samples may be missed. A sampling rate that is too low causes an artifact called aliasing. Digitisation paved the way for computer generated reporting.

When analogue signals are transformed to digital signals the analogue digital converter measures the voltage in reference to ground and then amplifies the signal by a known amount. The data is represented in a binary code, decimal code (ASCII value) or a Hex code (hexadecimal value). Examples of the different codes are given in table 11.1.

Table 11.1: Examples of how measured voltage is converted to a digitised code.

Measured analogue voltage (mV)	Amplified analogue voltage (V)	Binary code	Decimal code	Hex code
-2.0mV	0.0V	000000000000	0	0x0000
0.0mV	2.0V	100000000000	2048	0x0800
2.0mV	4.0V	111111111111	4095	0x0FFF

To achieve the best possible resolution (ECG quality) to view, print, manipulate or analyse the ECG, the higher the number of bits used to represent the information the higher the resolution. To the human eye when displayed on for instance a screen the difference between an 8 bit and 16 bit code may not be discernable, the difference is in the quality of the information when used for computerised automatic measurements and arrhythmia detection. To store the ECG the data must be compressed, then decompressed when the ECG is selected to retrieve without loss of data or distortion of the data. In 2002 the Food and Drug Agency (FDA) in the USA made it a requirement that all ECGs used in drug trials should be provided in a digitised XML format (eXtensible Markup Language). This was because the FDA had to examine hundreds of hardcopy ECGs to determine QT intervals in drugs trials and each had to be manually scanned to store them digitally (Brown and Badilini, 2009). The development of XML also provided the incentive and technology to move to digital storage in the general clinical environment. This has now largely superseded the practice of archiving paper copies other than in the patient's notes (Brown, 2005). In Europe a different system was developed called the SCP-ECG format.

Picture archiving and communication systems (PACS)

Regardless of the storage format used, the data must be placed into a database system which allows recall of individual patient records. The move has been towards PACS based storage which stands for picture archiving and communication systems. PACS allows not only image storage of all types from still to moving images, but also archiving of reports, rapid retrieval of information, retrieval of information at multiple sites at the same time, and manipulation of data. However, PACS systems use DIACOM for storage (Digital Imaging and Communications in Medicine) as it was originally developed to store X-ray, MRI and CT images which are best stored as pixelated raster files. It was not intended to store ECGs in either XML or SCP-ECG format.

This can be addressed by scanning the ECGs and uploading image files or converting to PDF files. A better solution is DIACOM-ECG which was developed to directly convert ECGs into a form including metadata that can be uploaded onto PACS systems, whilst support tools have been provided to convert XML and SCP-ECG files for DIACOM storage. Modern ECG machines contain several choices of storage format.

When choosing a PACS the following points should be considered:

- What will the ECG data be used for and does the system suit this purpose? e.g. is it purely for storage and retrieval, or will you need to analyse/reanalyse data, report on data at a different time, or transmit outside the department/practice?
- Can data be uploaded from all ECG machines in the department?
- When new technology including different storage formats become available can the equipment be updated and reconfigured?
- Are the data storage files compact in size and what is the memory capability? What happens if this is exceeded?
- Can the data be accessed from different computers or devices or are specialised devices required?
- Can data be annotated?
- Can patient identification be easily and fully removed e.g. for teaching and publication purposes?
- Can data still be manipulated for measurement purposes?
- What programming languages is the system compatible with?
- Can data be transmitted over the internet and can it be done in a safe encrypted manner?
- Can access to data be restricted? Can restriction be selective down to specific investigations?

Knowledge Discovery in Database

Now that large volumes of ECGs are being stored on PACS systems it is possible to collect this information onto even larger databases for furthering medical knowledge. Such systems are called Knowledge Discovery in Database systems or KDDs. The advantage of pooling information is that sufficient data is available to soundly statistically analyse from underrepresented populations and medical conditions for the first time. The main drawback at present is that ECGs stored in PACS come from many different sources, and are of varying degrees of quality.

Archiving digital records

Just as an ECG machine must comply with specifications to ensure the ECG obtained is not distorted the same process applies to archiving ECGs. The ECG data must be compressed for storage; this allows a greater number of ECGs to be stored. The methods used must protect the ECG fidelity.

1. Archiving on the electrocardiograph

Modern electrocardiographs all have storage capacity built into the device and can store around 100 ECGs. It is recommended that every ECG is stored to the ECG machine hard drive immediately after recording so that the process becomes routine and forms a part of the ECG recording process. Storing to the ECG hard drive requires only a simple push of a button or answering a prompt from the equipment.

2. Archiving onto a computer or PACS

It is recommended that data stored on the ECG is uploaded onto a departmental computer or archiving management system at the end of every session or at least at the end of every day. In departments where ECG recording volume is low this may be reduced to every couple of days or every week. Communication to allow data transfer is typically achieved through a USB storage device, removable media card, a modem, or LAN or wireless LAN connection. Access to both the hard drive on the ECG machine, departmental computers and data management systems must be password protected.

Transmitting ECGs for storage or remote interpretation

Because ECGs contain confidential patient data they must be transmitted securely. This typically involves the encryption of data before transmission. A copy should be archived by the individual who recorded the ECG according to normal protocol. The receiver may also archive a copy if agreement is made between centres.

Faxing ECGs

Some ECG machines have facsimile capability which allows the direct faxing of ECGs from the ECG machine to a remote fax receiver. Some of the drawbacks of faxing include:

- Sensitive information can be transmitted to the wrong fax number.
- The quality of the fax may be insufficient for the ECG to be clinically used or interpreted remotely, however an ECG faxed directly from an ECG machine produces better quality transmissions at the receiving end than one transmitted through a fax machine from a hardcopy.
- Gridlines sometimes do not transmit well; this can be overcome by photocopying the ECG first then faxing the photocopy.
- Someone needs to be close to the fax machine or there needs to be an alarm alert system in place.
- Faxes can be lost at the receiving end.
- If using in, for example, an ambulance situation using mobile phone technology (cell phone) reception can drop out only sending partial information or not be available at all.

Advantages of faxing include:

- If a second opinion is required or an interpretation the ECG can be seen by appropriate personnel for expert advice.
- The technique is fast.

e-fax or internet faxing

An e-fax is a fax sent via an e-mail attachment using a computer. This means you do not need a fax line or a fax machine to send or receive.

Digital ECG transmission

Digital ECG transmission followed on from faxing. It is available in most modern ECG machines and many defibrillators. The system is web based and uses the internet to transmit the ECG.

Summary of key points:

- Hardcopies of ECGs may be obtained using different writing systems. There are advantages and disadvantages to each, therefore when choosing an ECG machine the method of archiving in use should be carefully considered.

- It is anticipated that ECG hardcopies will be eventually replaced by digital archiving for viewing tracings

- ECG voltage signals are converted into digital codes for archiving. This is achieved by a digital converter which samples the ECG waveforms at a set frequency converting the voltages at the sample points to codes. There are different digital coding systems available.

- Hardcopy ECGs may be photocopied and faxed or mailed to another ward, department or facility. Digitally stored ECGs may be directly faxed from the ECG machine, e-mailed, or archived onto a PACS system or similar where they can be remotely accessed.

Key review questions

1. What are the advantages of digitising ECGs?

2. Can hardcopy ECGs be digitised?

References

Brown, B.D. (2005). 'The FDA's digital ECG initiative and its impact on clinical trials' in, Morganroth, J., Gussak, I. (Editors). *Cardiac Safety of Noncardiac Drugs: Practical Guidelines for Clinical Research and Drug Development*. New Jersey: Humana Press Inc. pp. 301–27.

Brown, B. D., Badilini, F. (2009). 'HL7 an ECG implementation guide.' Available at: http://www.amps-llc.com/website/documents/UsefulDocs/aECG_Implementation_Guide.pdf (Accessed 6/3/12)

Chapter 12
Introduction to quality control in ECG recording

By the end of this chapter you should be able to:

- appreciate the importance of quality control in ECG recording
- discuss the use of policies, guidelines and protocols
- understand the importance of calibration and calibration verification procedures
- appreciate the need to maintain records in relation to daily activity and routine maintenance.

The importance of quality control

Quality control is at the heart of recording an electrocardiogram. It is just as crucial for the ECG department with only one member of staff as it is for the world renowned ECG core research laboratory. Without quality control an ECG is useless and its interpretation pointless. If asked to produce quality control records for inspection many may struggle to do so. However aspects of quality control are performed regularly without thinking of them in these terms. This chapter should help the reader begin to recognise and appreciate the many aspects of quality control and ensure adherence to the basic requirements for recording electrocardiograms. It is important to realise that quality control is the responsibility of everyone. That includes managers, and those who actually use the equipment from permanent, to bank, locum and agency staff. Areas who train students should also be aware that students should be exposed to and involved in quality assurance processes right from the start of their training. It is about producing a careful, safe, alert practitioner who delivers an excellent diagnostic and patient care service.

Electrocardiographic quality control embraces many aspects you may not have considered including:

- ECG recording protocols
- correct calibration verification procedures
- inter-/intra-recording variability
- correct equipment management and record keeping
- ensuring correct and adequate training of all personnel and maintenance of continuing professional development
- recognition and elimination of artifact
- correct ECG electrode placement and lead attachment.

Some of these issues are discussed in their own chapters.

ECG recording policies, guidelines and protocols

The clinical environment must investigate, manage and treat all patients the same within a broad framework and based upon a hierarchy of evidence-based practice. This broad framework can be adapted for individual presenting symptoms, clinical findings and patient needs. The broad framework can be recorded primarily in written form for all staff to understand and implement in everyday practice. This occurs through the development of policies, guidelines and protocols. There are differences between these three possibilities but also large areas of overlap.

1. Policies

Policies are typically statements of stance on a particular key area. They define rules in the form of directives for example, 'it is the responsibility of all staff...'. Policies may be supported by protocols and guidelines. An example of a clinical policy would be an overarching infection control policy. Policies help to increase consistency in actions by increasing the possibility that different staff will act and make decisions in a similar manner.

2. Protocols

Protocols are a detailed set of instructions that must be followed in order to achieve the directives from a policy or a set of objectives. The combination of a policy and protocol into the one document is common. An example would be an ECG policy combined with a recording protocol. The policy section would outline circumstances when an ECG should be obtained, the protocol section would describe in detail how to perform an ECG. Overall protocols are more specific in detail than a policy and are in effect a ready reference guide or set of instructions for a particular area or investigation. Protocols may be written on a departmental basis but are more likely to be established in a hospital wide, trust or community wide setting, or research establishment to ensure continuity of care and standards. Protocols are also drawn up for individual research studies where electrocardiography is required.

3. Guidelines

A guideline is a set of statements which guide practice. Combined policies and guidelines are common.

ECG recording protocol

In practice most forms of ECG documentation in use are typically called protocols but when examined more closely are a combination of policy, protocol and guidelines in one. This makes sense as it is a general investigation performed by many different departments in many different clinical situations. For practice to be standardised everyone needs to be doing the same thing. Having an ECG recording protocol in place promotes high quality current best practice, provides a standard agreed set of 'when and how to do' instructions, and supports decision making when faced with non-standard clinical situations. Overall if well written and adhered to, protocols can improve patient care and cost efficiency. Protocols should be based upon current guidelines, evidence-based practice and research, and be regularly reviewed and updated. They are not intended to be set in stone forever and may challenge current traditional practice.

A typical protocol includes:

- a title page – title of protocol, date hospital, trust information etc.
- general information on the document itself – the author/s name and occupation, date of document, date for review and updating, the current version number, the department, trust or service etc., the protocol is designed for, any published guidelines on which the work is based, the name of the person or committee approving the protocol for use, and main distribution methods

- a contents page
- a background or rationale statement
- a definition of what an electrocardiogram is and its scope of clinical use
- a statement on professional guidelines, codes of conduct and proving competency
- a statement on minimal training requirements for staff
- reference to equipment required and any recommendations made
- a detailed set of instructions on how to perform the technique with a rationale for each step, this may require diagrams and figures for clarity
- links to related documentation – this may include existing protocols for hand hygiene, infection control policies
- unusual situations and adaptations
- references and additional sources of information.

Where departmental protocols exist these should contain all the relevant information described above but may in addition include specific instructions for use of the actual recording equipment available in the department and details of how the department processes its results and/or patients.

Positive reasons for having a protocol include the standardisation of a procedure, the research and inclusion of best practice, the sharing of knowledge and techniques across diverse settings and staff disciplines, providing transparency on procedures for all staff, and providing the opportunity to have procedures and practices challenged. A protocol may, where necessary, be adapted at an operator's own discretion or professional judgement, but only if this improves the care of the patient. Any deviation from the ECG protocol should be clearly annotated on the ECG obtained along with the reason why the deviation was necessary. The member of staff making the decision to alter the protocol for use on a single specific patient must be in a position to make an informed decision, be able to justify their action and fully understand the consequences of their action. For example, altering an ECG protocol to record in the seated position for a patient complaining of chest pain who is trapped in a car following a car accident is acceptable. To record an ECG seated in a chair because it is easier not to get a patient back into bed, it would take too long to get the patient back into bed, or it would require a hoist and two members of staff to get them back into bed is not acceptable. In fact to alter the ECG protocol in this situation would not only demonstrate clinical incompetence but if subsequent inappropriate action was taken regarding medication or further investigations based on the ECG findings then this would leave the operator open to a legal challenge. A protocol also clearly states in the case of a legal challenge, that suitable procedures are in place and helps inform risk assessment procedures.

Feedback on protocols should be actively sought and it is good practice to release a proposed protocol for a specified consultation period before finalisation and implementation. This provides the opportunity for staff to highlight ambiguous or incomplete sections, and inconsistencies.

Calibration and calibration verification procedures

Before measuring or interpreting any clinical data the operator must be sure that the equipment is working correctly otherwise the results will not be accurate and the interpretation will be flawed. It is crucial that the same machine settings are used throughout the world to allow comparisons to be made between patients, individual recording centres and countries. To achieve this calibration and calibration verification, also known as standardisation, is used.

Unfortunately the term calibration is often used interchangeably to mean calibration verification or standardisation. This has led to confusion over what the processes are and what the operator is actually doing when they check their equipment before use.

Calibration is the adjustment of a piece of equipment to produce a known output for a known input. Each component inside the ECG machine will have its own level of error within specified tolerance limits (the maximum and minimum values they are allowed to 'be out' by). When the components are all working together there is a total error which must meet specified standards of permitted variation tolerance for an ECG machine.

Calibration must be set for both voltage and time. Voltage is adjusted so that a one millivolt (mV) signal fed into the machine produces a deflection of 10mm on paper along the Y axis and a signal lasting for 0.2 seconds produces a tracing that lasts for 5mm on paper on the X axis. In almost all modern ECG machines this calibration setting cannot be changed although the ratio chosen for a specific recording can be altered temporarily. The heights of the ECG waveforms correspond to the voltage created in the body and therefore must be accurately reproduced to create a diagnostic quality ECG (Houghton and Grey, 2003).

Calibration verification or standardisation

Calibration verification or standardisation on the other hand is the process via which the equipment itself and/or the operator checks and confirms that the calibration set at manufacture has not changed i.e. drifted to a larger or smaller value in terms of voltage or speed. All equipment will drift over time due to simple environmental factors. These include aging of the components, changes in ambient temperature and humidity.

Operator performed calibration verification

Calibration verification or standardisation is the process performed when the operator checks the calibration signal to ensure the ECG has been correctly recorded and is suitable for clinical use. Everytime an ECG is recorded a calibration signal is also generated and a printout is produced typically at the beginning or end of the ECG tracing. This allows the operator to confirm that everything is satisfactory for clinical use. ECGs are recorded on graph paper but without calibration and calibration verification the values of the squares are meaningless. The operator should check every ECG to ensure that the calibration signal is 10mm tall and 5mm wide. If this criterion is not met than the machine cannot be adjusted by the operator and must be removed from use until it can be serviced or returned to the manufacturer.

ECG paper

ECG paper is a specialised type of graph paper divided by vertical and horizontal lines into large and small squares (Figure 12.1). The larger squares measure 5mm by 5mm, whilst the smaller squares measure 1mm by 1mm. With only this information the significance of the squares is not known. However when we calibrate and then verify the calibration we place a value on each of the squares in terms of height which represents millivolts on the vertical axis and width which represents time in seconds on the horizontal axis. Paper speed is also calibrated so that the paper moves at 25mm/second along the X axis. This speed is standard in the UK and US (Hand, 2002).

Providing the equipment is correctly calibrated at 25mm/second, the width of each large square (5mm) delineated by darker, thicker lines, will represent 0.2 seconds. Each of the smaller squares within the large square (1mm) will therefore represent 0.04 seconds. Again at the standard calibration of 1 millivolt (mV) = 10mm, the height of each large square (5mm) will represent 0.5mV. These figures are required to verify calibration and to perform waveform and interval measurements.

In general, when choosing ECG paper, the surface should be ultra smooth to avoid distorting the waveforms and to allow the paper to flow easily through the equipment. The graph lines should be accurately reproduced to ensure accuracy of voltage and timing measurements, but there are other quality control issues to consider too.

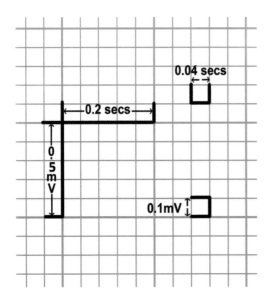

Figure 12.1: Standard ECG graph paper.

All ECGs machines are not designed to use the same type of paper and although a certain paper may work with the equipment its thickness or weight may affect the paper feed speed, its surface may not be designed for the recording medium used causing blurring and smudging, or it may not record at all in the case of a non thermal paper used in a thermal printer machine.

Some ECG papers are not stable, in other words the recordings made on them will fade or even disappear with time. Paper stability should be carefully considered to meet requirements for the minimum storage period of patient records in practice area. Where archiving over a specified period of time is required and particularly for research purposes, the choice of recording paper stability may be crucial for maintaining the quality of the tracings in a readable sharp condition. Other papers fade rapidly if placed inside plastic pockets (see chapter 12).

Many ECG papers are thermal and register a record of the ECG when exposed to heat. This may be achieved by a heated stylus in older machines or by a thermal array printer in more modern equipment. Quality control issues with thermal paper are many, but the most problematic is the accidental loss of data. Placing a chart on top of a radiator or on a sunny window sill can destroy the ECG. Likewise a carelessly placed coffee cup or chart placed over an equipment heat vent can do the same.

As a general rule of thumb source ECG paper from reputable manufacturers only who can guarantee precise standards,; cheap is not always best. Paper should be manufactured in specialist medical chart paper companies and a check should be made to ensure alternative papers meet or surpass the original equipment manufacturer specifications for paper to use with their equipment. Many companies are ISO certified manufacturers and will list the number of the ISO specifications they meet. This means that an organisation called the International Organisation for Standardisation has stated the manufacturing process is compliant with their standard.

Clinical tip

When choosing paper to ensure quality control consider:
- Thickness – is it suitable for the specific equipment?
- Surface smoothness – will it distort the ECG waveforms?
- Image stability – will the recordings last?
- Thermal sensitivity – will recordings accidentally be obliterated if exposed to heat?

Inter-/intra-recording variability

There is evidence to suggest that there is both inter- and intra-recording variability. Intra-variability occurs when the same operator records an ECG several times on the same patient. Inter-variability occurs when different operators record several ECGs on the same patient. These are changes introduced due to variation in technique and may mask or alter changes due to true physiological developments. Both inter- and intra-variability may be reduced by careful electrode placement. Where possible if serial ECGs are required for a specific reason, e.g. cardiac transplantation or clinical trials, the same operator should perform them all. In addition consideration should be given to marking the electrode positions on the chest. Keeping the same electrodes in place between recordings is not recommended as apart from sweating under the electrodes, and infection issues, the electrodes are prone to movement and slipping over time.

Equipment management and record keeping

ECG machines play a crucial role in the safe and accurate delivery of diagnostic data. Staff using the equipment and/or overseeing a department's management must be fully aware of how to ensure its continued safe condition and safe use.

Accurate, clear and easily accessible records are the key to effective equipment management and quality assurance processes. Records help to:

- quickly identify the stock of equipment available for use
- ensure prompt and well planned preventative maintenance measures, routine recalibration and rapid early repairs. Planned preventative maintenance should adhere to manufacturer recommendations
- provide a record of each piece of equipment location, supplier, purchase and replacement date
- provide an audit trail of maintenance procedures and servicing
- enable swift appropriate action to be taken in the case of a recall from the manufacturer or an alert from the Medical Devices Agency.

All equipment that is in storage and not in current use or equipment that is used infrequently must also be managed as above. A daily calibration log should be kept for each piece of equipment and stored with the servicing records. In addition a departmental log should be kept detailing each electrocardiogram recorded, indicating the patient, the electrocardiograph used, and the operator.

1. Routine maintenance by users

To keep machines in good working order practitioners must take responsibility for routine maintenance procedures. Measures should be in place to facilitate the detection and reporting of failure to work and visible defects in the equipment and/or recordings. This includes the regular checking of cables and connections for any damage or fraying, regular cleaning with a mild detergent solution, preparation for use and checking the equipment is working correctly through calibration verification assessments and through the examination of the quality of the ECG tracing produced. Defective and unsafe pieces of equipment should be immediately removed from use.

If equipment becomes contaminated, the decontamination procedures followed should meet both the infection control regulations in use and the manufacturer's instructions to prevent external and internal damage to the ECG equipment.

At the clinic:

Consider the requirements of a good routine maintenance record for an ECG machine:

- **What items do you want to check?**
- **How often should you check the identified items? On a daily, weekly, monthly or quarterly basis, maybe even on a yearly basis?**
- **How should you record the information?**
- **Do you need information to be signed off?**
- **If something goes wrong are your records sufficient to identify any emerging patterns?**

2 Medical Device Alerts

In the UK Medical device alerts are issued by the Medicines and Health Care Products Regulatory Agency. Typically MDAs are received by the purchasing department who alert the appropriate risk management staff, managers and where appropriate end users etc. The risk management team identifies the appropriate action to take after receiving an MDA. This may be the immediate removal of a piece of equipment, a change in operating instructions, or simply an alert to be aware of a certain finding. All actions outlined in the MDA must be followed, they are not optional. A copy of the MDA and action requirements must be filed in the medical equipment record file and any actions required logged in the equipment records.

- If an item is recalled, immediately remove from use, label clearly that device should not be used and follow instructions to return to manufacturer.

- If a device is to be treated as a hazard but not to be recalled remove from use, label clearly that device should not be used, follow handling instructions, do not return to use until notified it is safe to do so.

Warning

When replacing parts on an ECG machine such as broken patient cables, only use those recommended by the manufacturer. Some patient cables contain protection circuits and replacing these with a different model may put the patient and practitioner at risk.

Risk assessments

A risk assessment is simply part of good management and quality control. Under Health and Safety legislation (1974), staff have a duty of care to look after their own health and that of others who may come in contact with the ECG equipment. This encompasses the equipment, the process and the consumables. The risk assessment process identifies the hazards of recording an ECG and of having an ECG recorded. It then tries to minimise the risks from the identified hazard of causing a specified harm. In the case of the ECG machine, hazards would arise from the equipment being an electrical device.

On-going quality assurance checks

A specified percentage of ECGs recorded should be regularly checked by another member of staff for quality within a specified period of time. When a new staff member is learning to do ECGs this should be set at 100 per cent of the tracings immediately after recording. This allows quick identification of poor quality tracings and the opportunity to re-record immediately. It also provides a learning opportunity for the staff member to see exactly what is wrong with a tracing made and for them to understand that this is not acceptable clinically and needs to be of clinical quality for use. It also gets the staff member into the way of examining their ECG as it emerges from the machine and correcting any fault immediately.

The number of ECGs examined and the frequency of checking is adjusted as each staff member grows in experience and demonstrates awareness and competence in obtaining a high quality tracing every time.

Experienced members of staff of all grades should continue as part of departmental quality control methods to have a specified number of their ECGs examined by another member of staff at regular intervals.

Summary of key points:

• Quality control is a key component of an electrocardiographic service. It provides the mechanism to ensure that data is clinically useful.

• The development of policies, guidelines and protocols ensures a consistent, evidence-based approach to the performance of ECGs.

• Accurate calibration of equipment is fundamental to obtaining valid clinical data. Calibration should be confirmed on every ECG.

• A departmental log should be compiled for daily patient activity, routine calibration and maintenance. In the event of a medical alert specific machines and patients can be traced. In the event of a medical error evidence of the equipment's suitability for use can be accessed.

Key review questions

1. What are the advantages of a protocol written by committee rather than by an individual?

2. What are the possible complications of the paper speed being faster by 10%?

3. How would the error in question 2 be recognised?

References

Hand, H. (2002). 'Common cardiac arrhythmias.' *Nursing Standard.* **16**(28): 43–52.

Health and Safety at Work Act (1974) available from: http://www.legislation.gov.uk/ukpga/1974/37/contents (Accessed April 2012).

Houghton, A.R., Grey, D. (2003). *Making Sense of the ECG: A hands-on guide.* 2nd edn. Hodder Arnold: London.

Chapter 13

Infection control in ECG recording

By the end of this chapter you should be able to:
- define healthcare associated infections
- appreciate potential sources of infection during ECG recording
- recognise the importance of hand hygiene.

The settings in which ECGs are recorded vary throughout and within various countries. But regardless of where these tests are carried out, maintaining infection control is an important and integral part of the process.

Healthcare associated infection

Healthcare associated infection (HAI) is a term used to describe any infection occurring due to healthcare or contact with a healthcare setting. The incidence of HAI varies throughout the world. It has been estimated that up to 0.25 million HAIs are contracted in Canada annually (Zoutman *et al.*, 2003) and 1.7 million in the USA (Klevens *et al.*, 2007). The First European Communicable Disease Epidemiological Report (2007) estimated that in the region of 3 million HAIs occur each year in the European Union. However, the full extent of the global burden of HAIs remains unknown.

The immune system is responsible for protecting patients from infection. As the skin's physical barrier is one of the first lines of protection, any breach of this will increase the risk of infection developing. Practitioners will normally recognise if the skin barrier has been broken and take action to maintain infection control. In individuals with a suppressed immune response there is also an increased risk of developing an infection when exposed to a pathogen. Frequently many in this group may not be easily recognised, for example patients with an underlying disease, receiving radiation or taking drugs that suppress the immune system. Therefore it is necessary that infection control measures are taken at all times and not only when a risk is perceived.

Healthcare associated infection can result from any pathogen that is transferred in the healthcare setting. Although it is unlikely that healthcare associated infections could be completely eradicated by using an effective preventative strategy, many can be avoided. A number of clinical guidelines have been produced to help prevent and control infections in the healthcare setting. Practitioners have a responsibility to be aware of these guidelines and to implement them.

Potential Sources of Pathogens

There are numerous potential sources of pathogens in the clinical environment, however it is the hands of practitioners that frequently transfer pathogens between patients or from the surrounding environment to the patient. Many pathogenic sources have been associated with the areas that staff use in trying to prevent their spread. Sink taps have been implicated in a number of studies (French *et al.*, 2004; Griffith *et al.*, 2000) while Griffith and colleagues (2000) and Brooks and his co-workers (2002) have both indicated that soap dispensers can also be an infection source. Other areas that have also been shown to harbour pathogens include computer key boards (Schultz *et al.*, 2003), door handles (Barker *et al.*, 2004), staff identification badges (Kotsanas *et al.*, 2008), privacy curtains (Trillis *et al.*, 2008), medical records (Teng *et al.*, 2009) and tourniquets (Brennan *et al.*, 2009). Staff uniforms can become contaminated (Treakle *et al.*, 2009), however using a plastic apron can significantly reduce microbial contamination on the front of these (Babb *et al.*, 1983). The ECG lead wires have also been identified as a possible source and means of pathogen transfer (Jancin, 2004).

Pathogens can be transferred by direct or indirect methods. Direct transfer occurs when an infected host makes direct contact with the body of another host; this can occur between patients or between the practitioner and a patient. Indirect transfer occurs when the pathogen is transferred in some way other than by actual body to body contact. This transfer can occur via animate or inanimate mediators. Duckro and colleagues (2005) verified that vancomycin-resistant enterococci could transfer from intact skin or inanimate objects in the patient's room to the healthcare practitioner's hands and then be transferred to other surfaces. This provided a mechanism for the spread of pathogens throughout the healthcare environment. This study helped to confirm that a common route of indirect pathogen transmission via an animate mediator in the healthcare environment is the hands of the practitioner.

Hand hygiene

It is recognised that poor hand hygiene is a major contributing factor in the transmission of HCA infections. Studies by Pessoa-Silva *et al.*, (2004) and Pittet *et al.*, (1999) both demonstrated that high levels of hand contamination are associated with direct patient contact, while Pessoa-Silva *et al.* further established that gloves do not fully protect against contamination. The maintenance of good hand hygiene is therefore essential to reduce the pool of potential pathogens on hands and decrease the incidence of HAIs.

The potential scale of the HAI problem worldwide is so significant that the First Global Patient Safety Challenge 'Clean Care is Safer Care', one of the flagship programmes of the World Health Organization (WHO) World Alliance for Patient Safety, targets HAI (Pittet & Donaldson, 2005). The key element of this programme is hand hygiene (WHO, 2005). Pittet and co-workers (2006) described the five sequential steps required for indirect pathogen transmission by means of practitioner's hands:

- The pathogen must be present on the patient's skin or shed onto an inanimate object.
- When the practitioner touches the patient or the object, transfer to their hands must occur.
- The pathogen must be able to survive on the hands of the practitioner.
- Hand hygiene must be insufficient or omitted enabling pathogens remain on the hand/s.
- The contaminated hand/s must come into direct contact with the patient or an inanimate object that will come into direct contact with the patient so that transfer can occur.

Every working day the practitioner's hands will come into contact with a multitude of surfaces that are potentially colonised with pathogens. With each contact with a colonised surface a bidirectional exchange of pathogens will occur. Therefore it is essential that appropriate infection control methods are followed to prevent this transfer and the resulting spread of pathogens to patients and throughout the healthcare setting. As poor hand hygiene has been implicated as a major factor in the spread of HAI a source of guidance that reflects accepted best practices on hand hygiene has been published by the World Health Organization (WHO). The WHO Guidelines on Hand Hygiene in Health Care (2009) aim to promote a global improvement in hand hygiene; these guidelines promote the use of alcohol-based hand sanitation and the 'Five Moments for Hand Hygiene' model to indicate when hand hygiene should be performed (Sax *et al.*, 2007; WHO 2009). The five moments for hand hygiene are:

- prior to patient contact
- prior to an aseptic task
- following exposure to body fluids
- following patient contact
- following contact with the patient's surroundings.

By performing appropriate hand hygiene at the five key moments the transfer of pathogens can be interrupted and the risk of HAI reduced.

Practitioners must be able to decontaminate their hands when required. If hands are visibly soiled or the practitioner has been in contact with a patient with Clostridium difficile, diarrhoea or vomiting they will require washing, at other times the use of an alcohol-based decontaminant may be more appropriate. When using an alcohol-based hand product it must come into contact with all surfaces of the hands and be allowed to evaporate. Effective hand washing requires a number of steps. These include wetting both hands before applying the appropriate detergent. Rubbing the hands together to create a soapy lather following a recommended method such as the 'six step' technique. This will ensure that all surfaces are cleaned. Rubbing hands together briskly and for approximately 15 seconds at each of the six steps will assist in dislodging pathogens. Once the hands have been washed they should be rinsed thoroughly so that all soap residue is removed. Disposable paper towels should be used to dry the hands.

'Six Step' hand washing technique

Wet hands and using approximately 5ml of liquid soap perform a minimum of 5 backward and forward strokes in the following steps based on the standard Ayliffe technique (1978).

1. Place palms of the hands together and rub palm to palm working soap into a lather.
2. Place palm of right hand on back of left hand and rub. Repeat, swapping over with the palm of the left hand on the back of the right hand.
3. Rub palm to palm again but this time with the fingers interlaced so the sides of the fingers are being washed.
4. Using the fingertips of the right hand rub the palm of the left hand. Swap hands and repeat.
5. Rub the thumbs with a rotational movement and rub all parts of both hands well.
6. Rub backs of fingers with hands interlocked.

Rinse hands well and dry thoroughly wth a disposable paper towel.

Personal protective equipment

It is recommended that gloves are used when recording ECGs. Additional personal protective equipment should be used when a risk has been identified. This frequently involves the use of aprons and gloves. Disposable aprons and well-fitting gloves must be available for practitioners to use when necessary. Hands should be washed before and after the procedure. Local policies and procedures must be followed. When protective equipment is used it should be removed when the procedure is complete and the waste disposal policy followed.

At the clinic:

Review the departmental facilities for hand decontamination.

Is there an area where you can wash your hands?

How are the taps operated?

Where are the soap dispenser and paper towels positioned?

Are there any potential improvements to be made?

ECG Equipment as a Source of Pathogens

Reusable Welsh cup electrodes along with limb plates and straps are still available for purchase. Therefore it is surmised that these items are still used in the clinical setting. Reusable ECG electrodes and limb plates have been shown to pose a cross infection risk. In 1973 Lockey and colleagues reported that a patient acquired a Klebsiella aerogenes blood infection following cardiac by-pass surgery from ECG electrode pads moistened with saline. Later Cefai and Elliot (1988) found that all Welsh cup electrodes they sampled had been colonised by bacteria. In the same study they also established that Staphylococcus saprophyticus can survive in conductive gel for up to 36 hours and cross contamination can occur.

The main problem with reusable electrodes is that in order to eliminate the possibility of cross infection it is not sufficient to wipe, or even wash in soapy water between patients; a full cleaning and decontamination process is required. This is time consuming, requires chemicals hazardous to health to properly clean them, or the application of heat/steam for an extended period of time and a very large supply of non-disposable electrodes available to keep the service running whilst each set is returned for decontamination after single use.

Trend and his co-workers (1989) compared the effectiveness of different methods to clean reusable electrodes. The only method that was shown to be effective was heating the electrodes to 60°C for one hour. Other methods, including wiping the electrodes with tissues containing 70% isopropyl alcohol and immersing the electrodes in 70% ethyl alcohol at room temperature for ten minutes, were shown to be ineffective. As Welsh cup electrodes are designed to be reusable adequate cleaning between patients would not be possible in a busy healthcare setting.

Following an outbreak of Serratia marcescens, Sokalski and colleagues (1992) isolated Serratia marcescens with sensitivities identical to patient isolates from six reusable Welsh cup bulbs indicating that they were the possible source for the outbreak. With increasing awareness of infection control issues many practitioners have adopted the use of disposable ECG electrodes in an attempt to minimise the risks of HAI. However, evidence suggests that electrodes may not have been the only problem and that ECG leads also present a substantial risk for HAIs. Between June 1996 and July 1997 a burns unit experienced an outbreak of colonisation and infection caused by vancomycin-resistant Enterococci (VRE). During this outbreak 26 per cent of ECG leads tested cultured positive for VRE. Control measures including decontamination of the unit were carried out and it was thought that the VRE had been eradicated. All surveillance cultures had been negative for a five-week period when a routine culture from an ECG lead was positive. A culture taken from the patient on the same day was negative for VRE however three days later the patient had a positive culture. This culture had the same pattern of Pulsed-Field Gel Electrophoresis (PFGE) as the ECG lead and the last infected patient who had used the room 38 days previously (Falk *et al.*, 2000).

Further reports of contamination of cleaned and ready to use lead wires followed. In 2004 Jancin reported the key finding of a study carried out by Dr. Paul Brookmeyer of University of Wisconsin Hospital and Clinics, Madison. His research indicated that 77 per cent of cleaned ECG telemetry leads sampled were contaminated with one or more antibiotic-resistant pathogens. Termini and co-workers (2009) also examined the potential for cross infection due to ECG leads and presented their findings as a poster at the 2009 Annual Meeting of Tennessee Society of Anesthesiologists. As a minimum all leads were wiped with ammonium chloride solution and if used on a patient known to have MRSA 1/16 per cent bleach was also used. Cultures were obtained following cleaning, all cultures were positive. Albert and colleagues (2010) identified a large number of bacterial pathogens that could be cultured from cleaned reusable lead wires. They found that rates of contamination ranged from 49 to 80 per cent with bacterial growth in 62.8 per cent of the cultures. Fourteen of the bacterial species identified posed a risk or potential risk for human infection.

Infection Control and Electrocardiogram Monitoring

Because contaminated ECG lead wires provide a possible vehicle for cross infection their use in the clinical setting needs to be reviewed in relation to infection control. Current cleaning protocols appear to be ineffective in removing pathogenic contamination and therefore leave patients at risk of contracting a HAI. In many of the reported cases of cross contamination via ECG equipment when disposable single use electrodes and/or leads were used cross contamination ceased. These products can be expensive but this cost has to be considered in relation to the cost implications associated with an outbreak in your healthcare practice and the possible consequences for patients.

Warning

Always unplug the electrocardiograph from the mains power supply before cleaning.
Do not immerse any part of the electrocardiograph or cables in fluid.

Cleaning the electrocardiograph

Always follow the manufacturer's instructions in relation to cleaning and only use approved cleaning solutions.

In general all debris is removed from the electrocardiograph, the surfaces and leads are then wiped with a soft cloth that has been dampened with a solution of mild soap and water. Do not use abrasive cleaning materials or agents. Do not use strong solvents as these can damage the equipment. Once a surface has been wiped a soft clean dry cloth is used to dry it. Take care to ensure that moisture does not enter the main body or connector ports. The frame, storage compartments and wheels should all be cleaned regularly.

Summary of key points:

- Healthcare associated infections are a global problem and are caused by interaction with the healthcare system.

- There are numerous sources of infection, many are frequently overlooked. One such source is electrocardiography. Reusable electrodes have been identified as a potential infection source and as a result disposable electrodes are recommended.

- Good hand hygiene is the most effective method of reducing healthcare acquired infections.

Key review questions

1. When washing hands the use of a nail brush is not recommended, why?

2. When should infection control precautions be applied?

3. Why is it important that gloves are well fitting?

References

Albert, N.M., Hancock, K., Murray Y., Karafa, M., Runner J. C., Fowler, S.B., Nadeau, C.A., Rice, K.L., Kraiewski, S. (2010). 'Cleaned, ready-to-use, reusable electrocardiographic lead wires as a source of pathogenic microorganisms.' *American Journal of Critical Care* **19**(6): 73–80.

Aycliffe, G.A.J., Babb, J.R., Quiraishi, A.H. (1978). 'A test for hygienic hand disinfection.' *Journal of Clinical Pathology* **31**: 923.

Babb, J.R., Davies, J.G., Ayliffe, G.A.. (1983). 'Contamination of protective clothing and nurses' uniforms in an isolation ward.' *Journal of Hospital Infection* **4**(2): 149–57.

Barker, J., Vipond, I.B., Bloomfield, S.F. (2004). 'Effects of cleaning and disinfection in reducing the spread of Norovirus contamination via environmental surfaces.' *Journal of Hospital Infection* **58**(1): 42–9.

Brennan, S.A., Walls, R.J, Smyth, E., A., Mulla, T., O'Byrne, J.M. (2009), 'Tourniquets and exsanguinators: a potential source of infection in the orthopedic operating theater?' *Acta Orthopaedica.* **80**: 251–5.

Brooks, S.E., Walczak, M.A., Hameed, R. (2002). 'Chlorhexidine resistance in antibiotic-resistant bacteria isolated from the surfaces of dispensers of soap containing chlorhexidine.' *Infection Control and Hospital Epidemiology* **23**(11): 692–5.

Cefai, C., Elliot, T.S.J. (1988). 'Re-usable ECG electrodes – a vehicle for cross-infection?' *Journal of Hospital Infection* **12**(1): 65–70.

Duckro, A.N., Blorn, D.W., Lyle, E.A., Weinstein, R.A., Hayden, M.K. (2005). 'Transfer of vancomycin-resistant enterococci via health care worker hands.' *Archives of Internal Medicine.* **165**: 302–7.

European Centre for Disease Prevention and Control (2007). The First European Communicable Disease Epidemiological report. p1. Available at: www.ecdc.europa.eu/pdf/Epi_report_2007.pdf (Accessed 12.4.12).

Falk, P.S., Winnike, J., Woodmansee, C., Desai, M., Mayhall, C.G.(2000). 'Outbreak of vancomycin-resistant enterococci in a burn unit.' *Infection Control Hospital Epidemiology.* **21**(9): 575–82.

French, G.L., Otter, J.A., Shannon, K.P., Adams, N.M.T., Watling, D., Parks, M.J. (2004). 'Tackling contamination of the hospital environment by methicillin-resistant Staphylococcus aureus (MRSA): a comparison between conventional terminal cleaning and hydrogen peroxide vapour decontamination'. *Journal of Hospital Infection.* **57**: 31–7.

Griffith, C.J., Cooper, R.A., Gilmore, J., Davies, C., Lewis, M. (2000). 'An evaluation of hospital cleaning regimes and standards'. *Journal of Hospital Infection.* **45**(1): 19–28.

Griffiths, R., Fernandez, R., Halcomb, E. (2002). 'Reservoirs of MRSA in the acute hospital setting: A systematic review.' *Contemporary Nurse* **13**: 38–49.

Jancin, B. (2004). 'Antibiotic resistant pathogens found on 77% of ECG lead wires.' *Cardiology News.* **2**: 14.

Klevens, R.M., Edwards, J.R., Richards, C.L., Horan, T.C., Gaynes, R.P., Pollock, D.A., Cardo, D.M. (2007). 'Estimating health care-associated infections and deaths in U.S. hospitals, 2002.' *Public Health Reports* **122**(2): 160–66.

Kotsanas, D., Scott, C., Gillespie, E.E., Korman, T.M., Stuart, R.L. (2008). 'What's hanging around your neck? Pathogenic bacteria on identity badges and lanyards.' *Medical Journal of Australia.* **188**(1): 5–8.

Lockey, E., Parker, J., Casewell, M.W. (1973). 'Contamination of ECG electrode pads with Klebsiella and Pseudomonas species'. *British Medical Journal* **2**: 400–1.

Pessoa-Silva, C.L., Dharan, S., Hugonnet, S., Touveneau, S., Posfay-Barbe, K., Pfister, R., Pittet, D. (2004) 'Dynamics of bacterial hand contamination during routine neonatal care.' *Infection Control and Epidemiology.* **25**(3): 192–7.

Pittet, D., Dharan, S., Touveneau, S., Sauvan, V., Perneger, T. (1999). 'Bacterial contamination of the hands of hospital staff during routine patient care.' *Archives of Internal Medicine.* **159**(8): 821–6.

Pittet, D., Donaldson L. (2005). 'Clean care is safer care: a worldwide priority.' *Lancet* **366**: 1246–7.

Pittet, D., Allegranzi, B., Sax, H., Dharan, S., Pessoa-Silva, C.L., Donaldson, L., Boyce, J.M. (2006). 'Evidence-based model for hand transmission during patient care and the role of improved practices.' *Lancet Infectious Diseases*, **6**: 641–52.

Sax, H., Allegranzi, B., Uckay, I., Larson, E., Boyce, J., Pittet, D. (2007) 'My five moments for hand hygiene: a user-centred design approach to understand, train, monitor and report hand hygiene.' *Journal of Hospital Infection.* **67**: 9–21.

Schultz, M., Gill, J., Zubairi, S., Huber, R., Gordin, F. (2003). 'Bacterial contamination of computer keyboards in a teaching hospital.' *Infection Control and Hospital Epidemiology.* **24**(4): 302–303.

Sokalski, S.J., Jewell, M.A., Asmus-Shillington, A.C., Mulcahy, J., Segreti, J. (1992). 'An Outbreak of Serratia marcescens in 14 adult cardiac surgical patients associated with 12-lead electrocardiogram bulbs' *Archives of Internal Medicine.* **152**(4): 841–4.

Teng, S.O., Lee, W.S., Ou, T.Y., Hsieh, Y.C., Lee, W.C., Lin, Y.C. (2009) 'Bacterial contamination of patients' medical charts in a surgical ward and the intensive care unit: impact on nosocomial infections'. *Journal of Microbiology Immunology and Infection.* **42**(1): 86–91.

Termini, J., Epps, J., Bigge, J., Patteson, S.L. (2009). 'Potential for cross-infection with multi-use electrocardiogram lead wires'. Poster Presentation at: 2009 Annual Meeting of Tennessee Society of Anesthesiologists; Nashville, TN. Available from: http://www.asaabstracts.com/strands/asaabstracts/abstract.htm;jsessionid = 256OEA3842FAAOC123117A4BOB34D686?year = 2009&index = 8&absnum = 22 [Accessed March 2012].

Treakle, A.M., Thom, K.A., Foruno, J.P., Strauss, S.M., Harris, A.D., Perencevich, E.N. (2009). 'Bacterial contamination of health care workers' white coats.' *American Journal of Infection Control.* **37**(2): 101–5.

Trend, V., Hale, A.D., Elliot, T.S.J. (1989). 'Are ECG Welsh cup electrodes effectively cleaned?' *Journal of Hospital Infection.* **14**: 325–31.

Trillis, F., Eckstein, E.C., Budavich, R., Pultz, M.J., Donskey, C.J. (2008). 'Contamination of hospital curtains with healthcare-associated pathogens.' *Infection Control and Hospital Epidemiology.* **29**(11): 1074–6.

World Health Organization (2005). 'World Alliance for Patient Safety. Global Patient Safety Challenge 2005–2006. Clean Care is Safer Care'. Geneva: World Health Organization. Available at: http://www.who.int/patientsafety/events/05/global_challenge/.../index.html [Accessed April 2012].

World Health Organization (2009). 'Guidelines on Hand Hygiene in Health Care. First Global Patient Safety Challenge: Clean Care is Safer Care'. Geneva: World Health Organization. Available at:www.chp.gov.uk/files/pdf/who_ier_psp_200907_eng.pdf [Accessed April 2012].

Zoutman, D.E., Ford, D.B., Bryce, E., Gourdeau, M., Herbert, G., Henderson, E., Paton, S. (2003). 'The state of infection surveillance and control in Canadian acute care hospitals.' *American Journal of Infection Control* **31**(5): 266–73.

Chapter 14
Training and continuing professional development

By the end of this chapter you should be able to:
- understand the need for suitable ECG recording training
- demonstrate an awareness of training support methods
- recognise the need for continuing professional development
- evaluate the use of audit forms to identify learning needs
- define learning needs and set appropriate goals.

Training in ECG recording

Lack of training or poor training is responsible for the majority of correctable faults seen in ECG. Examples include artifactual ECGs, use of inappropriate filter settings, missing or incomplete patient data and missing explanations for alterations in standard technique etc. It is also responsible for largely undetectable but present faults in the finished ECG such as misplaced precordial chest electrodes. Training should not be the often used 'see one, do one, teach one' kind. It should be in-depth, of adequate length, be primarily hands-on not theoretical, include an assessment of technique and logbook of performance, and be ongoing on a yearly basis.

There is no formalised requirement for training in ECG recording. However all practitioners should only work within their capabilities and within their professional codes of conduct. These codes require that staff are adequately trained and undergo suitable continuing professional development (CPD) training in all areas in which they practice. A period of supervised apprenticeship by a competent experienced staff member is crucial and should last for a specified agreed period. A training logbook and practical assessment is good practice and forms a record of basic training. The concept of minimal numbers of ECGs recorded on an annual basis to maintain competency should also be considered.

A more formalised method of training is to work towards taking a nationally recognised and respected examination. This proves that the practitioner has undergone the minimal theoretical and practical training considered appropriate to record ECGs in accordance with safe and responsible working practices. The Society for Cardiological Science and Technology offer a Proficiency in Electrocardiography Certificate to all healthcare staff. These examinations include both a practical ECG recording examination and a multiple choice paper. A number of other training programmes will meet the same learning outcomes.

Further details and syllabi for the SCST examinations in Electrocardiography may be obtained from the Society's website at http://www.scst.org.uk or from EBS (SCST), Suite 4, Sovereign House, 22 Gate Lane, Boldmere, Sutton Coldfield, B73 5TT, Telephone: 0845 838 6037, E-mail: admin@scst. org.uk.

The supervised training period

Training should be supervised by a qualified member of staff and provide a safe and open environment for learning. Training ideally starts on volunteers and only progresses to real patients after the rudimentary aspects of skin preparation and electrode placement have been learnt. As the student progresses in skill and confidence, they move from observation, to practicing supervised, then to remote supervision and finally to recording ECGs alone. A senior member of staff should be available to offer assistance even when the student is ready to record on their own.

Support for training

Simulated training sessions with either computer software or manikins aid learning and reinforce practical training sessions on real patients. The student should be introduced to a wide range of patients and learn to use different electrocardiographs and recording formats. Although there is a wide range of training packages available for interpreting ECGs it is more difficult to access materials for recording ECGs. Many clips and sites on the internet contain misinformation and great care should be taken if using web sources with students. Engagement with realistic scenarios enables students to identify with the applicable clinical situations and develop skills that help them succeed. Simulation develops student confidence and results in higher levels of efficiency and consistency (Sinclair and Ferguson, 2009).

Staff with competency problems

If a staff member appears to be having difficulties achieving the set competencies for using electrocardiographic equipment an action plan to assist should be formulated between the trainer and the staff member. It would be usual practice to keep a record of the agreed training plan and any alterations required in the staff member's personal file. Where a difficulty in competency is noted:

- identify any barriers to effective learning e.g. noise, too small control panel, restricted space, not enough time to learn fully etc.
- arrange a more suitable environment for training or alter existing environment
- observe the person using the equipment to gather insight as to where assistance may be required
- break down the skill into smaller steps
- encourage progress no matter how small
- encourage the continued practice of the technique
- consider using another staff member with a different teaching approach to support the learner.

Training content

Practical and theoretical training cannot be successfully separated for electrocardiography. Therefore an integrated approach to training is best. Students should become familiar with all aspects of recording including the necessary patient care, ECG recording technique, anatomy, physics and instrumentation.

Continuing professional development

Practitioners are required to maintain continuing competence in all aspects of work that fall within their scope of practice. Professional organisations often have established programmes that support its members in this area. In many cases this will be by keeping a continuing professional development portfolio. Evidence for portfolios is obtained from a range of sources including reflection on practice, feedback from peer observation and attendance at courses. For electrocardiography, the first step with regard to assessing CPD needs requires the practitioner to assess themselves against practice standards. An audit can be used for this purpose and an example is shown in table 14.1.

Table 14.1: Example CPD requirement audit form.

Electrocardiography CPD audit to identify learning needs	
Has the professional been assessed within the last year recording an ECG?	Yes ☐ No ☐ If no carry out a formal observation
Has the practitioner undertaken update training in ECG recording in the last year?	Yes ☐ No ☐
How many ECGs does the individual record per month?	
How many ECGs are recorded in the immediate practice area per month?	
Has the individual undertaken a recognised formal ECG examination?	Yes ☐ No ☐
What area/s do/does the practitioner feel they need updating in or training in?	
Does the practitioner have responsibility for supervising or training other practitioners in recording ECGs?	Yes ☐ No ☐

If the practitioner has not been assessed recording an ECG within the last year they should proceed to peer observation. This is carried out by a suitably qualified, competent and updated colleague in electrocardiography. Feedback from this observation will provide insight to aspects of practice that the practitioner currently does not have awareness of. Reflection on the self-assessment and feedback from the peer observation are key to identifying the individual's learning needs.

Table 14.2: Example ECG observation audit.

ECG observation audit	
Task	**Comments from reviewer**
Was patient greeted and the test explained appropriately?	
Was adequate patient ID obtained?	
Was suitable consent obtained?	
Was patient dignity maintained?	

cont.

141

Was patient positioned in the supine position or the need for a semi Fowler position appropriately assessed?	
Was the skin adequately prepared?	
Was a method of electrode location used?	
Were the correct anatomical positions for the limbs and precordial electrodes attained?	
Was the correct colour code used?	
Were the patient details checked before entering into the computer	
Was a good quality ECG obtained?	
Was calibration and paper speed checked?	
If relevant was any artifact eliminated?	
Was the filter setting checked and was a notch filter used?	
Was the ECG annotated if required?	
Was patient informed of details for obtaining results?	

Identifying learning needs

Identifying learning needs can sometimes be straightforward, for example if there has been a change to a role with new responsibilities. At other times it is more difficult, especially when seeking out weaknesses in knowledge and skills. Identifying learning needs that are unknown to the professional is very difficult and normally requires a peer review process. Time invested in identifying areas that require development in order to maintain competence is well spent as it prevents undertaking CPD activity that is not relevant to current needs. Areas can also be addressed to meet future aspirations in relation to career progression. When new knowledge and skills are applied in the clinical environment learning has taken place. Attendance at a training course is not the same as learning. Learning needs in ECG can be identified by comparing performance against evidence-based guidelines and other sources of best practice such as audits and peer reviews.

Once learning needs and the CPD audit shortfalls have been identified, a learning plan should be completed. The learning plan should clearly state the learning need/goal, how these will be met, outcomes/indicators of success and a timeframe for completion/review. It is vital to evaluate new learning as a result of attaining the identified learning goals. In particular how this has impacted on practice and if additional training is required.

Table 14.3: Example learning plan form.

Learning needs identified:			
Action Plan:			
Learning Need	How this will be met	Review date	Outcome

Summary of key points:

- It takes considerable skill to record an accurate ECG. Therefore a structured approach to training is required.

- There are numerous ways to support ECG training. The method used should be tailored to the student's individual learning needs.

- Training is not a one-off event and it is the responsibility of the practitioner to identify their on-going learning needs.

- The use of audit forms provides a structured approach to identifying gaps in knowledge and skills. Once learning needs have been identified clear goals should be established along with a plan of how to attain the goals.

Key review questions

1. What are the barriers to undertaking continuing professional development?

2. Who benefits from CPD?

3. Evidence suggests that although CPD is strong amongst the workforce, few maintain their CPD documentation. What are the consequences of not keeping portfolios and other documentation up to date?

References

Sinclair, B., Ferguson, K. (2009). 'Integrating simulated teaching/learning strategies in undergraduate nursing education.' *International Journal of Nursing Education Scholarship* **6**(1) Article 7.

The Society for Cardiological Science and Technology and the British Cardiovascular Society (2010). 'Clinical guidelines by consensus: recording a standard 12-lead ECG an approved methodology.,
Available at: http://www.scst.org.uk/resources/consensus_guideline_for_recording_a_12_lead_ecg_Rev_072010b.pdf (Accessed 6/3/12)

Answers to key review questions

Chapter 1

1. There are few absolute contraindications to recording an ECG as the technique is noninvasive, painless, relatively quick and simple for the patient. Performing an ECG does not cause harm and makes a valuable contribution to the overall diagnosis when interpreted in conjunction with other clinical information.

2. There are normally no clinical implications of measuring different heart rates from two consecutive ECGs. This is because there is normal daily variation in the heart rate as it is affected by stress, infection, temperature, medications and exertion immediately before the recording etc. However unexplained significant increases or decreases in heart rate are clinically important.

3. Modifiable inaccuracy is one that is typically introduced by the recording equipment or the practitioner recording the ECG. It can include placing the electrodes on the incorrect anatomical positions, or not correctly preparing the skin which introduces artifact into the recording. Modifiable inaccuracy can be limited by good technique and following standardised ECG recording guidelines. A non-modifiable inaccuracy is usually introduced by the patient themselves or is an inherent problem with the recording equipment. Non-modifiable inaccuracy includes pronounced chest movement effort with difficult breathing in for example chronic obstructive pulmonary disease. Whilst this inaccuracy cannot generally be eliminated it may in some cases be reduced.

4. Factors that may contribute to intra-individual variability in the ECG include precordial and limb electrode variation, the presence of artifact, respiration patterns, pregnancy, weight changes and position of patient other than supine etc.

Chapter 2

1. The first rib is obscured by the clavicle and the twelfth rib is predominantly covered by muscle therefore increasing the chances of making an error in identifying the adjacent intercostal spaces.

2. In most individuals it is easier to locate the angle of Louis and count from the second intercostal space found just below it, than locating the ribs and spaces using any other method. Unless there has been previous surgery or trauma to the sternum the angle of Louis method is less prone to making a mistake in its location. Although the angle of Louis may be located at the level of the third intercostal space this is an extremely rare occurrence.

3. In this specific case using the swab method would prove problematic as the wiring of the sternum post-surgery had left a number of bumps in the sternum which would have affected the swab angles. Also the angle of Louis may have changed position. Therefore other techniques that identify the rib spaces not using the sternum could be used.

Chapter 3

1. When recording a standard 12-lead ECG you should do nothing, the electrodes have specific locations which should be used. Bone, congested lungs, excess fatty tissue, pericardial and pleural effusions can all attenuate ECG signals. The point is that the ECG is standardised by keeping the electrodes in the same place every time it is recorded. In this way ECG abnormalities and changes over time can be identified and compared.

2. None in the 12-lead ECG. Texts frequently mix up instructions for monitoring ECGs with recording 12-lead ECGs. Muscles can cause an artifact in the ECG called somatic muscle artifact or muscle tremor (page 86). This can be very apparent in monitoring (or exercise ECGs) as the patient moves freely. However 12-lead ECGs are recorded at rest and the practitioner should have the necessary experience to recognise and reduce muscle artifact.

3. In theory there is no reason why not to use the fingers and toes. However, it is difficult to ensure complete stillness in fingers and toes and there are a number to choose from so standardisation would be difficult.

4. The first rib runs under the clavicle at the midclavicular line. Therefore another technique is to locate the midclavicular line and palpate vertically downwards. This initially tracks the first rib and will feel relatively hard. Then suddenly the fingers feel a springier region which is the second intercostal space. Palpating down the midclavicular line misses the first intercostal space altogether so spaces cannot be confused. From here it is simply a matter of counting on down the ribs and rib spaces. There is however only one recommended method which is the angle of Louis; other techniques are useful when the angle of Louis is difficult to locate or as a double check.

Chapter 4

1. Providing that the electrodes could adhere well to the skin, sweat actually improves ECG quality. This is because sweat contains electrolytes such as sodium and chloride. It is also moist therefore this combination reduces electrical impedance.

2. When a razor is use to remove hair this frequently results in skin irritation (razor burn). As skin is frequently cleansed with an alcohol-based product stinging and increased irritation may result. It is also possible to accidently remove the tops of small moles, skin tags and pimples. This increases the risk of infection in the area. During hair regrowth in-growing hairs (pseudofolliculitis barbae) may be a problem.

3. The stratum lucidum is a thin layer of dead skin cells. But it is only found in areas of thick skin such as the palms of the hands and the soles of the feet where it protects the lower levels from friction. It is not found in any of the areas where the ECG electrodes are placed.

Chapter 5

1. Electrodes should be small to be accurately positioned. This is particularly important if using electrodes which incorporate an adhesive ring as these can be very large making it difficult to position the electrodes on the chest without overlapping.

2. Examine the area to determine if the welts are the electrolyte gel, the adhesive ring or both. This gives information as to which part of the product is causing the problem. A few patients are allergic or sensitive to products in the glue used in the electrodes or chemicals used in the electrolyte. The risk of allergy/sensitivity increases if the skin has been damaged. Over-enthusiastic skin preparation can cause tiny breaks in the skin allowing the chemical to enter deeper than they normally would have. This can be a particular problem in the elderly where the skin may be thinner or dryer. If the area of irritation is much greater than the electrode size it could be that a component of the skin preparation is involved in the adverse reaction. If the patient is exhibiting an allergic reaction or sensitivity they should be seen by a physician before leaving the department to determine if treatment with a topical antihistamine or steroid is required. It can be useful to carefully wash the affected areas with water and pat dry. Inform manufacturer of problem and complete a complaints form if available. It is useful to send a sample of electrodes from the same batch back to the manufacturer so that any fault in the electrode can be tested for. Photographs may also be useful.

3. No for a number of reasons. Electrodes designed for children often have a milder chemical composition as children's skins are prone to sensitivity. Paediatric electrodes contain less adhesive and are therefore less likely to damage delicate skin when removed. In addition paediatric solid gel electrodes are smaller and fit the chest without overlapping.

4. An ideal electrolyte should have the following properties:

- highly conductive
- hypoallergenic and bacteriostatic
- does not dry out quickly
- is of a consistency that does not run
- water soluble for ease of removal
- non-staining.

Chapter 6

1. Because only lead I and III are affected this suggests there is a problem somewhere in the limb lead/electrode system. These are both Einthoven leads therefore using knowledge of lead derivation we know that lead I is the potential difference between the right and left arm, lead II between the right arm and left leg and lead III between the left arm and left leg. Therefore it follows that the common factor is the left arm. As a result, the electrode, the connection to the lead and the lead integrity should be checked.

2. When attaching the limb leads three of the colours used are common between the European and American colour coded system, red, black and green. However these are not attached to the same electrodes, for example red is attached to the right arm in the European system and the left leg in the American system. Therefore there is the potential for a serious error. In addition, because the remaining lead in the American system is white the practitioner could inadvertently think this is due to the lead being replaced due to breakage with a non-colour coded lead. Four of the six precordial leads are identical. The remaining two V4 and V5 are different so a problem should occur only with these two leads. However if the limb leads are incorrectly attached the ECG overall is of no value.

3. Rearranging the way the ECG is presented could result in misdiagnosis as changes between recordings might be mistaken as pathological. This could be addressed by clearly informing all personnel of the change via training days and strategically placing information relating to the changeover. It may also be possible to have the service engineer put a text box highlighting the change on the printout.

Chapter 7

1. The common-mode rejection ratio (CMRR) measures the ability of an amplifier to obtain the difference between two inputs while rejecting the signal.

2. The American Heart Association has set this limit as there is a potential for a patient to come into contact with any part of the electrocardiograph while at the same time being earthed through another pathway. To reduce the risk of this resulting in a fatal event the limit for leakage current has been set at 10 microamperes.

3. The ECG would be distorted and this could result in misdiagnosis.

Chapter 8

1. The key points should include:
- Use terminology the patient will understand.
- It is a painless procedure and records the electrical impulses generated by the heart.
- It is necessary to remove all clothing to the waist and expose skin on the lower limbs.
- The patient will lie flat throughout the procedure.
- The rib spaces will need to be located, this requires counting down the patient's chest.
- The skin will need to be prepared on the chest and limbs plus details of skin preparation.
- Electrodes will be placed on the prepared skin and leads attached to these.
- It is important to relax and remain still during the recording.
- The process will take 10 to 15 minutes.

2. It is important because many patients will be very anxious and concerned as to why they need an ECG, what will happen and what implication the results will have. As to obtaining good quality ECG, the patient has to be relaxed; a calm confident practitioner can help reassure the patient.

3. Once the electrocardiogram is removed from the electrocardiograph there is no way of confirming that it belongs to the patient therefore a name must be present. An incorrect age could lead to incorrect interpretation. Not including the time and date invalidates its use for future comparison. Failing to annotate any changes from standard will also prevent future comparisons.

Chapter 9

1. 1mA of current is not a fixed value. Some females may detect the tingle sensation as low as 0.7mA. There is actually a range between which most individuals detect the effects of electrical current; this is between 1 and –5mA. The value of detection also falls with damp skin and sweating, a common occurrence in the clinical situation, and with the use of electrode gel.

2. The electromagnetic interference resembles atrial fibrillation/atrial flutter. As EMI artifact is not well recognised it is frequently misdiagnosed as other clinical conditions and could result in inappropriate treatment. However on careful inspection P waves are clearly identifiable and the artifact continues throughout the QRS and T waves.

3. In a normal ECG the R waves increase in size from V1 to V2, therefore when reversed V1 has a larger R wave than V2.

Chapter 10

1. As the leads are acquired simultaneously comparisons can be made in relation to the waveforms in the same set of beats. Artifact will be seen as random activity in one or more leads and can then be disregarded in the analysis. However if artifact is present in all or the majority of the leads this will be interpreted as an arrhythmia.

2. The primary benefit of oversampling is the detection of narrow pacemaker spikes. Oversampling also improves signal quality at the high frequency cut off, i.e. it reproduces the sharp QRS and pacing spikes better.

3. As the input is the same the report could be different if the signals were processed by different methods. Signal processing can cause slight alterations in the signal, these may be significant enough to affect the interpretation.

Chapter 11

1. Some advantages of ECG digitisation include:

- the original can be preserved indefinitely in as good quality as when the tracing was originally made
- data can be shared remotely and quickly
- access to ECG data can be secured
- measurements made are more accurate
- fulfils research requirements
- saves paper and storage space.

2. Yes, hardcopy ECGs may be sent to specialised companies to digitise or can be completed by using a high resolution scanner and computer.

Chapter 12

1. The committee will have a number of members with different experiences and viewpoints. They can support the development of the document by providing constructive criticism and ideas so that the final work will be more acceptable to a broader audience. The time element involved in writing and the responsibility can be shared.

2. The heart rate will appear slower although this may not be a significant problem when measured in beats per minute. The significant problem is that the waveforms of the ECG will be slurred and intervals and durations will be increased, possibly resulting in misdiagnosis. An individual who is at the upper limits of normal QRS duration will most likely become just abnormal.

3. The calibration signal would be 5.5mm wide, this equates to duration of 0.22 seconds.

Chapter 13

1. A nail brush is not recommended because it can cause small abrasions that can provide a route for pathogens to enter the body. It can also cause skin to become dry and dry skin is more prone to infection.

2. They should be applied at all times within the healthcare setting. This is necessary to ensure that the possibility of health acquired infection is reduced.

3. Gloves should fit well, mainly to avoid interference with dexterity. But they will also reduce excessive sweating and muscle fatigue in the fingers. Gloves that are loose around the wrists pose a threat of hand contamination.

Chapter 14

1. Barriers to CPD include heavy workloads, limited time outside work, access to suitable CPD activities, costs.

2. Everyone benefits, the practitioner will be more confident in their role, the patient benefits from enhanced skills and the employer benefits from having an appropriately trained workforce.

3. If CPD documentation is not kept up to date problems can arise if selected to take part in an audit, the information is requested from the professional body and if a move in employment is available. As the documentation is required, pulling this information together at short notice will not reflect the depth of experience gained over the previous two to three years.

Index